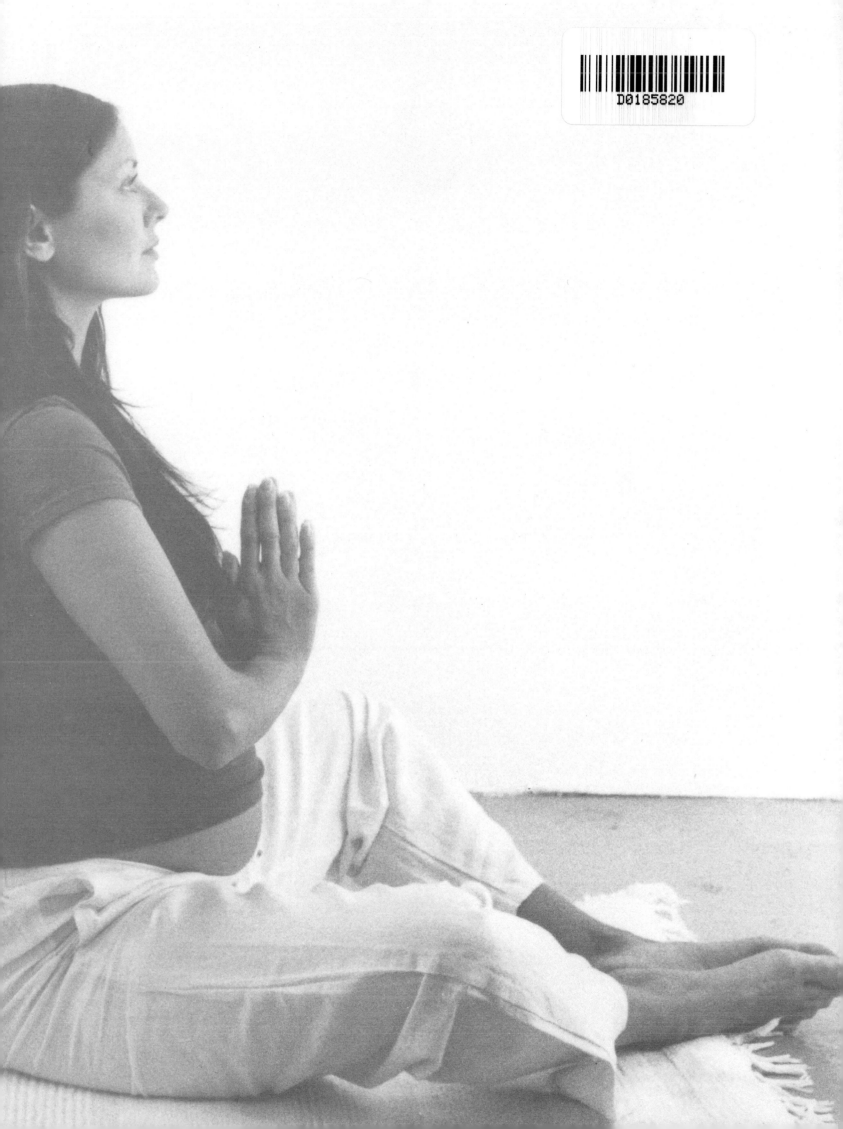

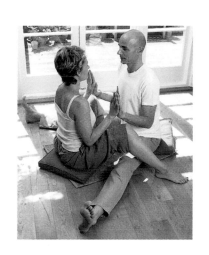

Prenatal

Yoga

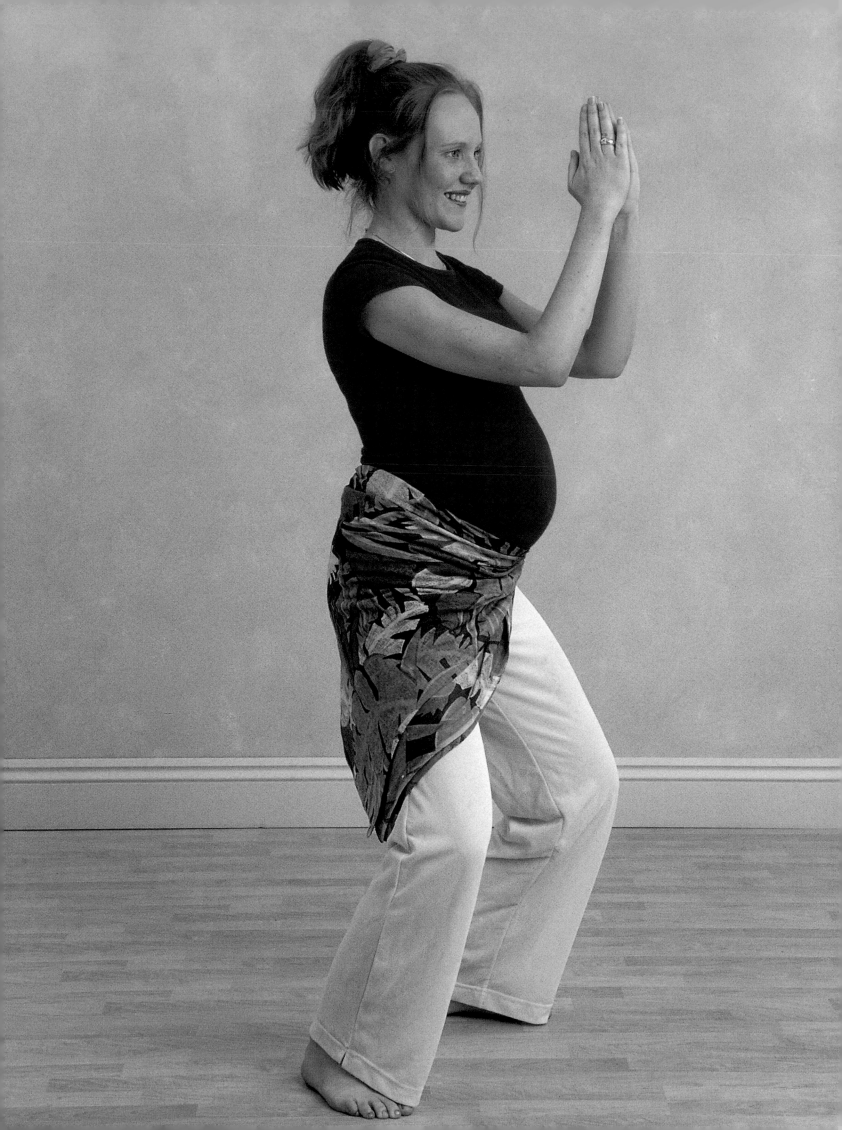

Prenatal Yoga

for conception, pregnancy *and* birth

doriel hall

françoise barbira freedman

photography by **alistair hughes**

LORENZ BOOKS

For Joanna and all babies who have a tough start, yet smile through life

This edition is published by Lorenz Books

Lorenz Books is an imprint of Anness Publishing Ltd, Hermes House, 88–89 Blackfriars Road, London SE1 8HA
tel. 020 7401 2077; fax 020 7633 9499
www.lorenzbooks.com; info@anness.com

© Anness Publishing Ltd 2002

This edition distributed in the UK by Aurum Press Ltd, tel. 020 7637 3225; fax 020 7580 2469

This edition distributed in the USA by National Book Network
tel. 301 459 3366; fax 301 459 1705; www.nbnbooks.com

This edition distributed in Australia by Pan Macmillan Australia, Level 18, St Martins Tower, 31 Market St, Sydney,
NSW 2000; tel. 1300 135 113; fax 1300 135 103; email customer.service@macmillan.com.au

This edition distributed in New Zealand by David Bateman Ltd, tel. (09) 415 7664; fax (09) 415 8892

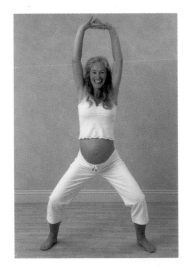

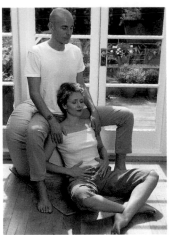

A CIP catalogue record for this book is available from the British Library.

Publisher: **Joanna Lorenz**
Project Editors: **Debra Mayhew, Ann Kay**
Photographer: **Alistair Hughes** Stylist: **Sue Duckworth**
Editorial Reader: **Jonathan Marshall**

Managing Editor: **Helen Sudell**
Designer: **Lisa Tai**
Illustrator: **Samantha Elmhurst**
Production Controller: **Claire Rae**

10 9 8 7 6 5 4 3 2 1

Publisher's note:
The reader should not regard the recommendations, ideas and techniques expressed and described
in this book as substitutes for the advice of a qualified medical practitioner or other qualified
professional. Any use to which the recommendations, ideas and techniques are put is at the
reader's sole discretion and risk.

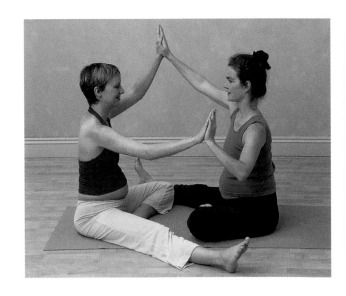

Contents

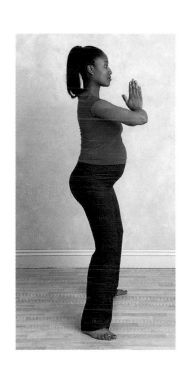

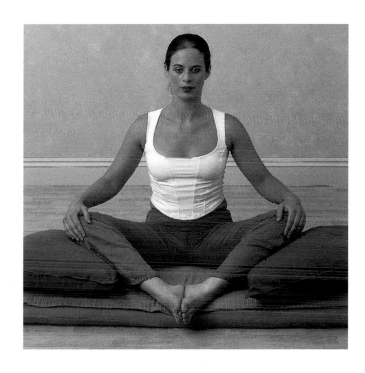

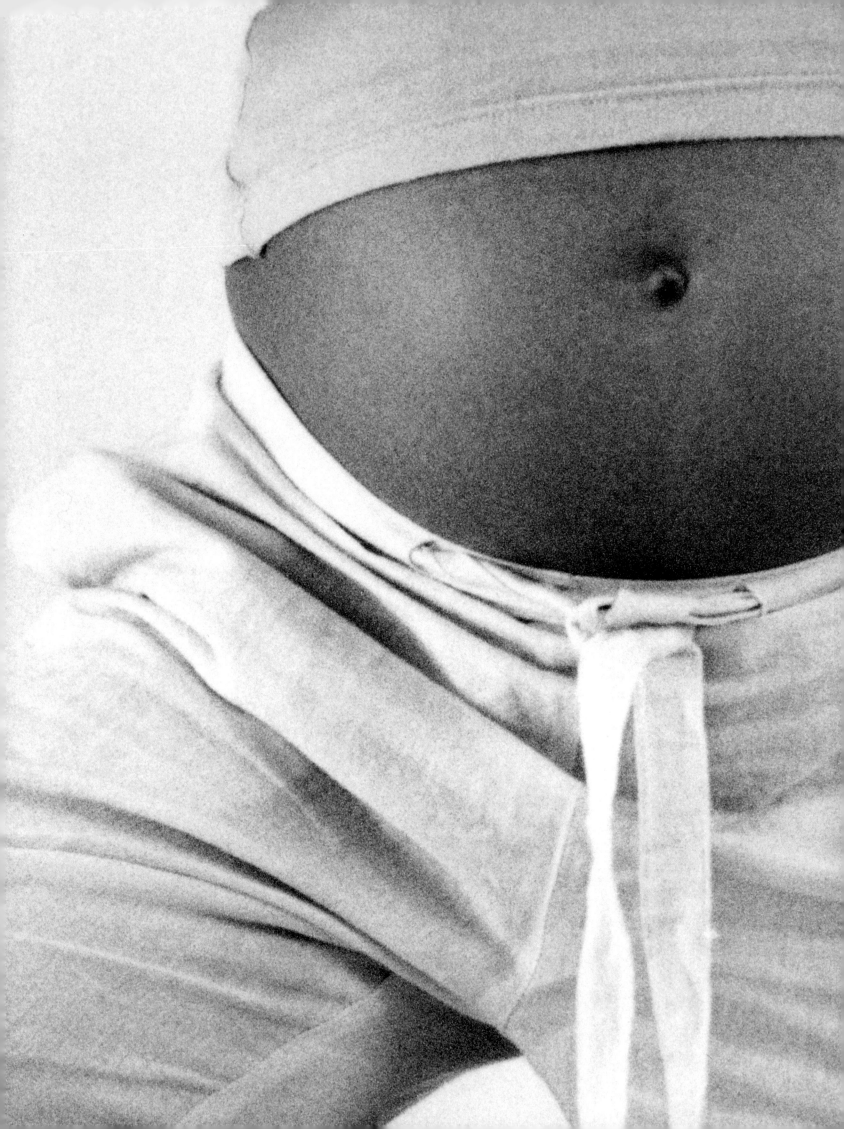

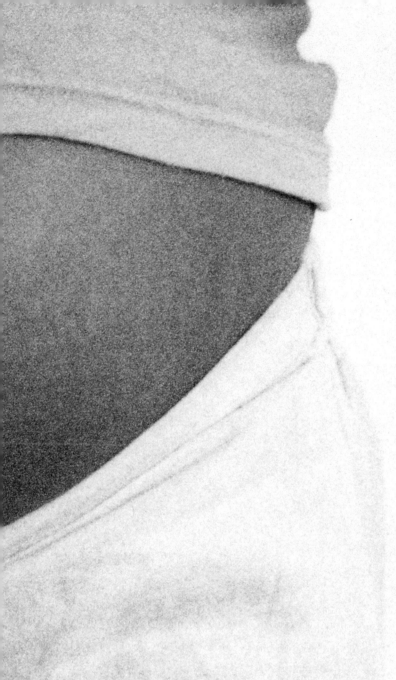

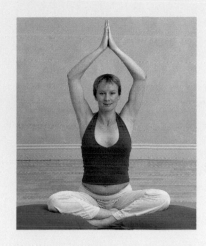

introducing
yoga

Yoga is a holistic life practice that will

greatly help you to enjoy your pregnancy,

right from conception through to the

birth. The specially adapted exercises in this

book are easy to follow, and a pleasure to

perform, whether or not you have ever

done yoga before. They will increase your

vitality, reduce your stress levels and make

you feel close to your growing baby long

before he or she is born.

Why yoga is the best form of exercise for you

Today, women have much more choice about when, and if, they conceive. Yet conception is still a mysterious and unpredictable event that has much to do with our personal well-being and mental outlook.

how yoga will help you

Regular yoga practice can help enormously, bringing you to a physical, emotional and mental peak. Strong, supple, focused, relaxed and happy, a woman such as this will be well placed both to conceive and to carry her baby joyfully right through to the birth – provided this is what she wants and there are no major medical obstacles.

Conception and pregnancy bring great changes. First there are the hormonal ones. Then there are the mental and emotional changes involved in altering your life so you can focus on the joy of motherhood and your baby's needs. Yoga can help you sail through these changes with a light step, a happy heart and a clear mind.

The yogic routines in this book are specially adapted to suit your needs, whether you are trying to conceive or are pregnant. They are easy to follow, and have been designed with your safety, and that of your baby, as the first priority. If you feel

uncomfortable with any exercise, don't persevere. Trust your instincts: deep self-awareness is the essence of yoga. There is plenty of choice throughout the book and the exercises are designed to make you feel great – at work, at home, anywhere.

a new way of being

• Feel well in yourself, with energy and enthusiasm for life, despite the hormonal changes and the inevitable anxiety. Yoga will ease the emotional tensions that can cause physical blocks – aiding conception, and also helping you cope serenely with the pregnancy.

• Be present in the moment – yoga is based on the practice of awareness, of living in the here and now. As you stretch and breathe and relax you will be living more fully than you ever could without this yogic awareness. Desiring and creating a baby is a wonderful experience. So make the most of every moment and enjoy it.

• Relate more deeply to those you love. Because yoga focuses on relaxation and breathing it opens our hearts to those around us, so that we draw them into our sphere of harmony and contentment. Your partner will appreciate being part of preparing for conception, enjoying pregnancy and giving birth. Friends, too, can enjoy practising yoga with you, while you prepare for conception and through your pregnancy. Above all, your unborn baby will bask in your love as the

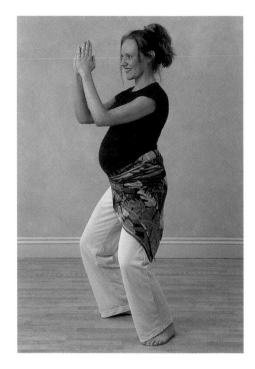

△ **Pregnant and happy. Regular and carefully adapted yoga practice gives you a light step and a light heart.**

foundations are established for a strong bond of love between you.

• Become more self-aware. You will find that you are constantly observing how you sit, stand, walk, breathe and relate to those around you, and that you are making subtle adjustments where needed. Change is cumulative – you will be amazed at the subtle changes you find in yourself.

• Become more fully who you are, as you become more relaxed and supple in body, mind, emotions and spirit.

▽ **Do not overstretch yourself when practising yoga. Here are three possible variations of the Dog Pose (see also 19). All are equally beneficial, as long as you do the one that is right for you.**

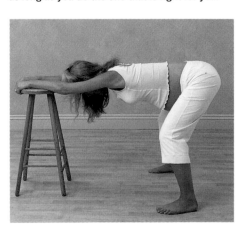

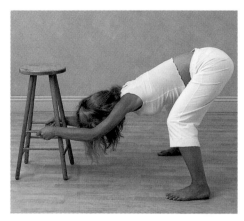

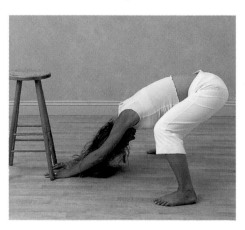

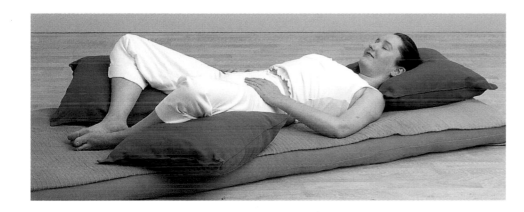

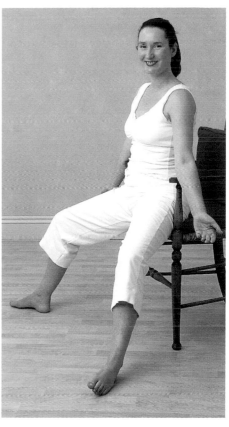

◁ ▽ To aid conception, yoga poses such as these two positions (below and left) make space for the baby by opening up the hips.

•You can do this kind of yoga at any age, at any time, anywhere, every day of your life. You will gain most with regular practice, but even a small amount is beneficial.

tailoring yoga to suit your needs

Yoga is infinitely adaptable – provided it remains holistic and no element is left out, and the principles of classical yoga that have been followed for millenia are respected. If the exercises are done without attention to breathing or the rhythm between activity and relaxation, they simply become "keep fit". This can, of course, be beneficial, but yoga gives you so much more. It creates a wonderful sense of deep-down well-being as well as increasing physical fitness.

how this book is organized

This book is divided into sections, each of which is tailored to a specific stage, and relevant aspects of your well-being:

Conception The emphasis at this time is on relaxing and opening up (physically and emotionally), and drawing energies into the Life Chakras in the abdominal cavity. This is where the reproductive system and its energies are situated. Movement, breath and relaxation are all practised in gentle ways.

Weeks 1–14 of your pregnancy The focus is on self-nurture and resting your body and mind as much as possible. This is to allow the vast hormonal changes that occur in early pregnancy to become established. There is only a little movement but plenty of breathing and relaxation.

Weeks 15–30 of your pregnancy The emphasis during these middle weeks is on a vigorous, happy enjoyment of life and your pregnancy and living from moment to

moment. There are plenty of loosening and strengthening exercises, co-ordinated by breathing, and interspersed with short rests and longer relaxations.

Weeks 31 plus of your pregnancy The focus at this time quite naturally falls on preparing for the birth. There is a greater use of props to help movement become as easy as possible and the all-important relaxation more comfortable, and a lot of breathing too. There are ways for your partner to help and so become fully involved in this incredible process, which also helps them to understand exactly what is happening.

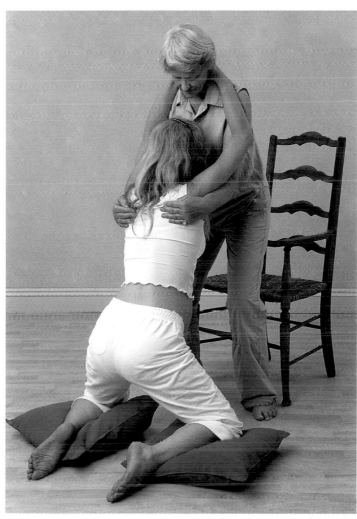

◁ During the last few weeks of pregnancy, yoga helps you to get in training for the birth. Here, a friend and a chair are used for support while practising birthing positions.

How yoga works for you

Yoga is a holistic discipline so it benefits you at every level, not only the physical one. Yoga philosophy maintains that a human being operates at several well-defined levels.

the five levels

There are five principal levels in yoga, and these are as follows.

Physical structure This includes bones, joints, muscles, skin and internal organs. Yoga develops physical strength, stamina and suppleness but these qualities are also developed at mental and emotional levels. Movement and posture are key elements.

Life processes This is the working of all the bodily systems, such as the respiratory and

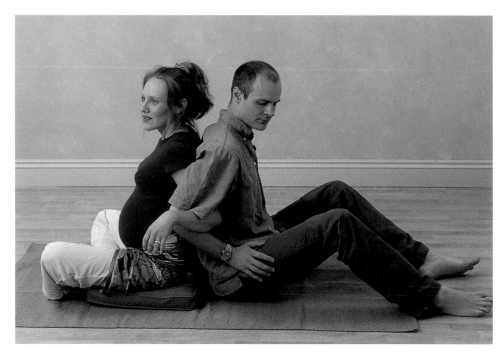

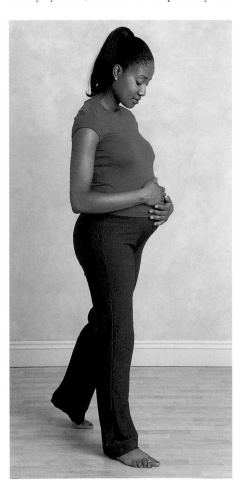

△ **Take time to relax and commune with your baby. This Walking Meditation (29) will help you to focus on the most important things in your life.**

cardiovascular systems, the various branches of the nervous system, the hormonal system, the digestive system and, of course, the reproductive system that will first create your baby and then support it in the womb. Breathing is the key element.

Internal organization This governs the workings of the brain and nervous system, so that all other body systems get the energy they need to do their jobs, just when they need it. In this way, internal harmony (also known as homeostasis) is sustained and we enjoy a state of contented well-being. Relaxation is the key element.

Clarity of mind This involves the ability to sort out our priorities, to concentrate on just one subject at a time until we are ready to turn our attention to another, rather than being too easily distracted by conflicting demands. In this way, we use our energy in a focused fashion, alternating periods of activity with those of relaxation. Being aware of posture, breathing and relaxation, and bringing them together in yoga practice, is a form of meditation, and meditation is a key element here.

△ **Yogic stretching, relaxing and unwinding with your partner helps you open up to each other.**

Emotions and deepest desires Yoga differentiates between automatic reactions and considered responses. We choose to respond warmly and positively to life rather than spin from one knee-jerk reaction to another. In this way, we take control of our lives and cultivate qualities of the heart. We develop mental stamina, plus emotional as well as physical suppleness and strength. Taking time and trouble to make a resolution that is meaningful for us, and confirming it while in deep relaxation, helps us to live more fully as the person that we choose to be – truly living our choices.

the Chakras

In simple terms, the Chakras are the points where the five levels of being, already described, meet and work together to produce the person that we are. The Chakras correspond to nerve plexuses along the spine in the physical body, and yoga aims to bring them into balance with each other in order to keep us healthy, happy and growing in wisdom and serenity.

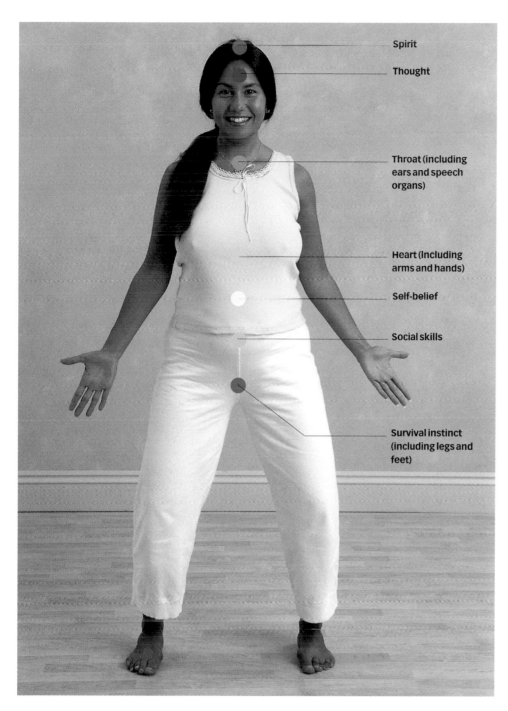

Spirit

Thought

Throat (including ears and speech organs)

Heart (Including arms and hands)

Self-belief

Social skills

Survival instinct (including legs and feet)

◁ The position of the Chakras in the human body. These fall into three main areas: the Life area (waist to toes), the Love area (chest and throat), and the Light area (head).

Love energies The two Chakras in the chest area are concerned with relationship, or Love energies. The heart is often called the "organ of feeling", and we express those feelings through the voice box in the throat. How we breathe profoundly influences our nervous system, which in turn determines to a large extent how we are feeling in ourselves and towards other people. Breathing with awareness could be said to be the heart of yoga, as all the other practices are linked with the movements of our breath. Relaxed breathing and deep relaxation practices allow us to open our hearts in welcome to all those beings we interact with, as well as to ourselves.

Light energies The two Chakras in the head are concerned with our mental, or Light, energies. It is these that sustain the clarity of our thought processes, our powers of observation and awareness, our focus on the job in hand, our choices and our decision-making. Practices that work with focus, awareness and meditation are all exercising our Light Chakras.

All yoga practices help to harmonize the energies of the Chakras and to maximize their combined energies.

Life energies The three Chakras in the abdominal cavity are concerned with vitality or Life energies. These include the energies that operate in the reproductive system to prepare for, conceive and create a baby, and the energies in the digestive system that nourish the body (and fetus) and clear away the waste products. These systems all lie in the abdominal cavity. Quite a lot of our prenatal yoga practice is aimed at enhancing vitality, to facilitate conception and later to make more space in the abdominal area as the baby grows larger. We also focus on the spinal and pelvic muscles that hold the reproductive organs in place and on bringing vitality to the whole reproductive system.

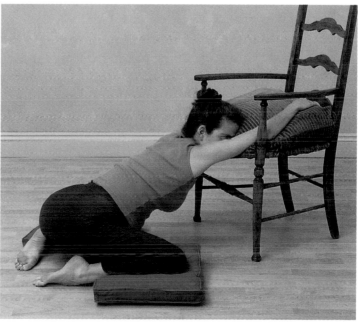

◁ Spinal stretching for alignment is always an important part of yoga practice as it encourages the flow of energy through the Chakras. This aspect needs special attention during pregnancy as the body shape and weight are constantly changing.

opening your body and your self

Whether you are trying to conceive or are already pregnant, it is vital to remain open at all levels. A woman is probably at her most welcoming at this time, offering her love, her body, her womb, her breasts, her nurturing ability, her home and her whole self as a safe haven. This openness is the pinnacle of femininity – and no experience could be more feminine than welcoming and nurturing the baby growing in your womb. Yoga for conception and pregnancy focuses on staying open and creating more space – more space in the lower abdomen for the baby, more space for the digestive organs to process the food needed by mother and baby, more space for the lungs to provide oxygen for mother and baby.

letting energy flow freely

Openness is a yielding, welcoming quality, but it is not a shapeless "giving in", nor a collapse, for it is literally backed-up by the strength and support of the spine. A key focus in yoga for both conception and pregnancy is to increase and maintain the alignment of the spinal and pelvic bones in order to provide free flow of vital energies and to protect the growing baby. This is vital for several reasons:

• To enable all the systems of the body to perform their functions without pressure or congestion. This is especially important when you are planning to conceive.

"Open the window in the centre of your chest and let spirit move in and out."

Rumi

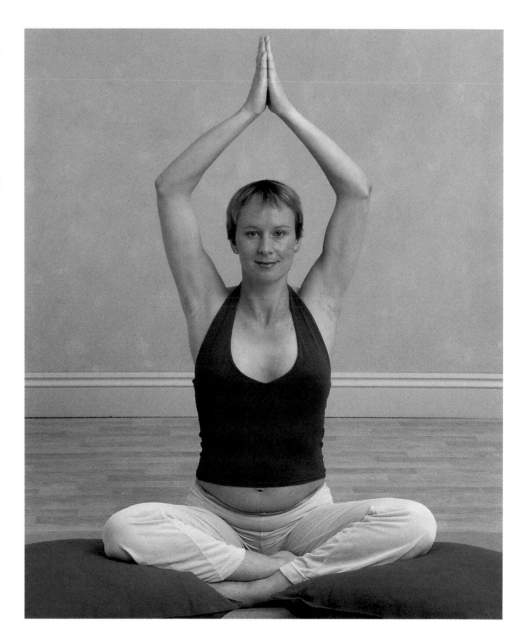

△ **In many poses, cushions placed under the knees protect your ligaments from undue strain.**

• To hold the baby in place, to create space for movement as he or she develops, and to make room for vital nourishment to pass through the placenta to the baby without any hindrance.

• To allow free passage through the spine of energies that activate the Chakras, as well as the mechanisms that are vital for the smooth running of the nervous system.

All our bones are held in place by muscles and ligaments. Muscles need to be exercised in order to remain strong and flexible and to have the stamina to go on doing their job for as long as necessary. Muscles that are not exercised at first become stiff and then atrophy, which can lead to greater fat deposits. The muscles that support our body's weight are the biggest and strongest ones. In classical yoga, we exercise them a great deal by doing standing poses where the weight of the trunk is taken by gravity through the legs and feet, which are firmly planted on the floor. In pregnancy, however, movement and rhythm are introduced to avoid the strain of holding

THE THREE MAIN STAGES OF PREGNANCY

Here you can see how the spine changes shape and the organs get increasingly squashed. Yoga helps to keep the organs working well and strengthens the all-important, supportive spine.

At 8 weeks

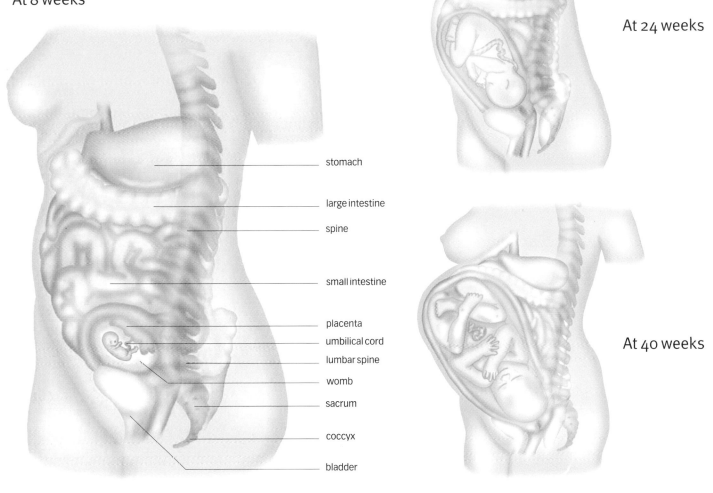

stomach

large intestine

spine

small intestine

placenta

umbilical cord

lumbar spine

womb

sacrum

coccyx

bladder

At 24 weeks

At 40 weeks

the classical positions. Various supports may also be used, to avoid tiring or straining while standing. Many poses are performed either sitting down (less tiring than standing) or lying down (where gravity works with you and the ground supports you).

posture and breathing

Yoga creates a virtuous circle whereby the more you become aware of good posture and alignment of the spine, the more you will pull yourself up whenever you notice you are drooping. The more you stand tall, the better you will breathe and the more vitality you will have. The more vitality you have, the less you will droop and the more you will naturally stand well and move with a spring in your step. Yoga is a holistic discipline, so improvement in any area affects all other areas for the better.

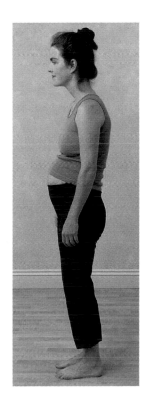

◁ Poor posture can spark all kinds of problems. Compression of the spine leads to pain in the neck and upper back as well as the lower back, while poor breathing from congestion of the lung space inevitably contributes to tiredness and low vitality. Slack abdominal and pelvic muscles lead to congestion in the abdomen and possibly lower back pain and swollen ankles.

▷ Good posture means that your head and neck are erect and balanced between the shoulders, and your spine and pelvis are properly aligned. Your abdominal and pelvic muscles are strong enough to support the baby and your chest is open so that the breathing muscles perform fully and fill the body with a positive vitality. Finally, your legs are strong, springy and balanced.

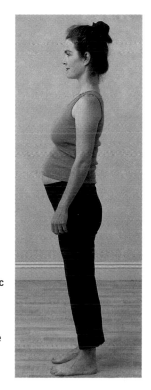

How to get the most out of your yoga

It is better to practise yoga for a few minutes each day than not at all. Some days it may only be possible to stretch your spine while standing in the kitchen waiting for a kettle to boil, or to practise your breathing at your desk after a prolonged spell on the telephone or computer. Do, however, find a quiet space and the time to practise whenever you can, daily if possible. When you use a particular place for yoga, a wonderful atmosphere builds up. Your yoga corner welcomes you and surrounds you with peace and safety, so you immediately relax, and this makes your yoga session a deeply fulfilling experience. Anywhere quiet and comfortable is suitable. Adorn it with flowers, pictures and other things that make you feel happy, and you will soon transform it into your personal haven.

getting started

You will probably find most of the equipment for your yoga practice around your home. A list of handy items follows.

• A yoga mat, or a similar-sized piece of non-slip carpet, to practise on.

• Several cushions, large and small – to put, for example, behind your back or under your head or knees.

• A beanbag to lean against.

• A variety of seats at different heights to sit on or place a foot on.

• A firm, upright chair for breathing exercises and meditation.

• A tape recorder and tapes to make your own recordings for deep relaxation.

• A light rug or blanket to cover yourself during relaxations.

• Several surfaces to push or pull against, such as a wall or a kitchen counter.

deep relaxation

Relaxation is a key practice in yoga and should not be omitted, whether you rest completely after each sequence of movements or practise deep relaxation at another time in the day. Ideally you should do both, so that you learn how to switch off at will. By restoring the natural rhythm of activity and rest in your life, you restore the body's natural balance. To do this, you need to alternate exertion, which achieves short-

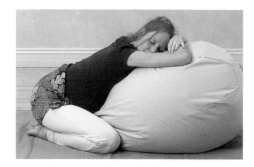

△ **Achieving a deeply relaxed state is a key element in good yoga practice. Help this along with cushioned supports and soothing tapes.**

term benefits, with the rest needed to achieve long-term benefits. These benefits include good digestion, repair of bodily tissues, release of stress, communication with your own inner world (meditation), and balancing and realigning the energies of body, mind, emotions and spirit.

The structure of your relaxation will depend on whether it is to last 10, 15 or 20 minutes. Many people make an audiotape to guide them in and out of their relaxation. This means that you can relax without worrying about missing out any parts of the session or overrunning. It is a really good idea to make several tapes, varying in length, to cover any eventuality. Whether you are making your own tape or not, be guided by the relaxation suggestions that follow.

a tailor-made relaxation session

During this session, you will plant a positive thought-seed deep into your mind, so think carefully beforehand what it is to be. No one can create this for you because it arises from deep within you but affirmations might include, "I feel ready to conceive", "I am enjoying my pregnancy", "I feel confident and happy about becoming a mother", and "life is wonderful". The affirmation should

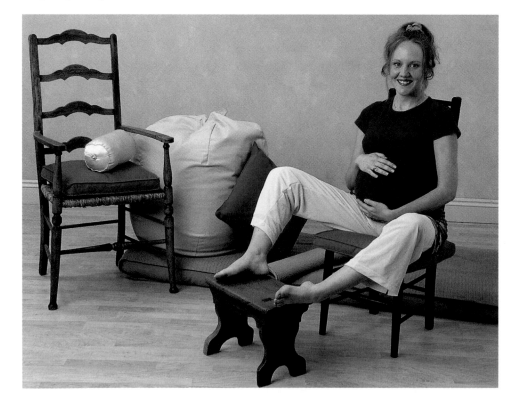

◁ **You don't need special, expensive equipment to practise yoga. Choose props that will support you so that you can be as comfortable and relaxed as possible.**

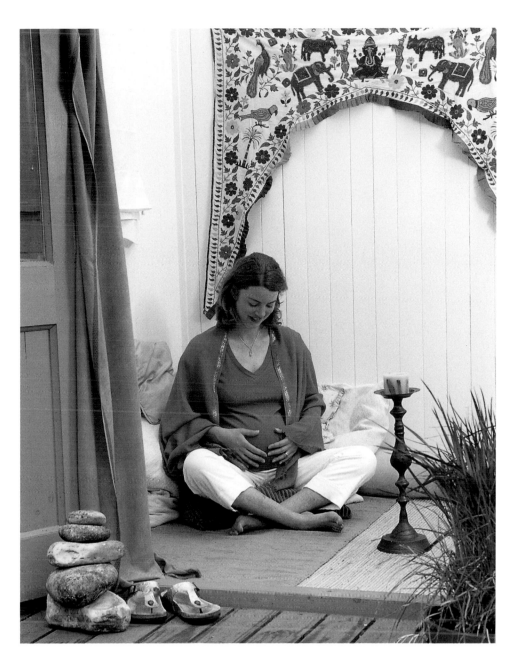

▷ A meditation corner filled with peaceful and beautiful vibrations is an ideal setting for yoga, and anyone can set up a simple corner at home.

address any doubts or fears you may have and help to dissolve them. Such positive affirmations are extremely powerful, especially when repeated daily while in a state of deep relaxation. Gradually, it will replace any negative seed-thoughts that you may have been harbouring for years, perhaps since early childhood. Just let go and forget about this early conditioning, for you are an adult now, ready and able to choose for yourself how you wish to be.

Experiment to find your most comfortable position (remember that this will change as your pregnancy advances), with cushions for support where appropriate. Now either switch on your tape or start to run mentally through these instructions, in this order:

• Take your focused attention to every part of your body, especially hips, shoulders, neck and face, to check that it is comfortable and relaxed. Wherever you find tension, breathe out deeply into that area to release the blockage.

• When your body is settled, turn your attention to your breath. Watch the process of breathing, how the air comes in through your nose cool and dry and moves right down into your lungs. How it then

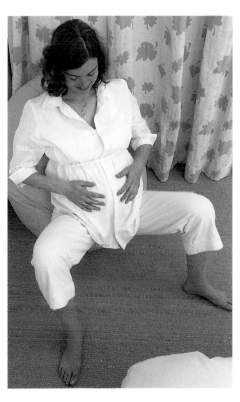

changes its quality and feels warm and moist as it is breathed out. Focus on your breathing for a few moments.

• Breathe into your heart space, building up feelings of welcoming love for the baby that you hope will come, or has already come, into your womb.

• If you are already pregnant, move your attention to the baby growing within you and delight in its presence in your life. Tell your baby of your joy, and feel how he or she is responding to your love and nurturing attention.

• While you are feeling deeply relaxed, open and receptive, repeat your seed-thought to yourself three times, slowly and clearly, so

◁ You may wish to vary where you do your yoga sessions – perhaps doing breathing or relaxation practices in one spot, and exercises in another.

that it takes root and grows in your mind and in your heart.

Now, instruct yourself to come out of the relaxation slowly, reversing the sequence with which you went in, but moving through it much faster.

• Tell your baby or hoped-for baby of your complete love.

• Return your attention to your breath and watch its flow. Then start to expand your breathing to wake up your body slowly. Your eyes will open automatically when your breathing has woken you up.

• To start bringing movement to your body, move ankles, wrists and neck gently. Now have several good, long stretches, yawning or sighing with long breaths out.

• Roll on to your side before coming up on to all fours. Rock your pelvis a little before getting up slowly.

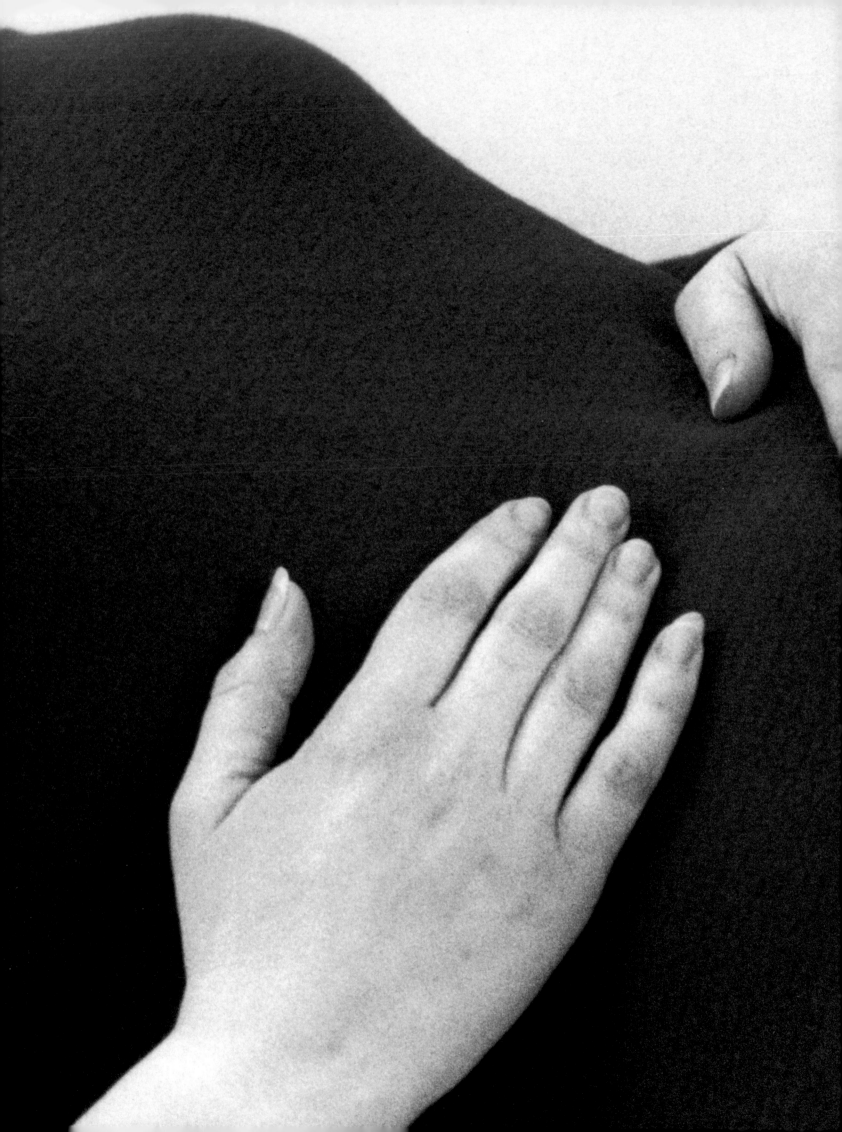

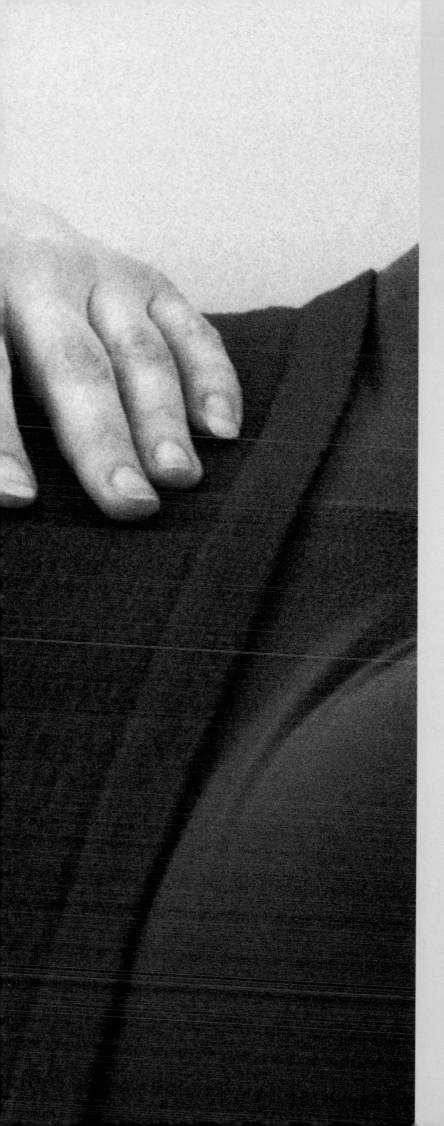

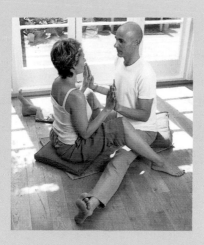

healthy
conception

Conception is a miracle of energy,

timing and receptivity. These qualities are

enhanced through regular yoga practice,

which improves the smooth functioning

of the reproductive system. Then, when a

ripe ovum (egg) is claimed by an eager

sperm and slips into the prepared, waiting

womb, the two will fuse into one and a

unique new person can grow within the

nurturing embrace of the mother's body.

How yoga can help you conceive

Stress can impede conception because it ties up so much of our vital energy – and this is detrimental. If stress is claiming energy for keeping our muscles uptight, our minds on overload and our emotions all churned up, the other systems of the body have to manage on the energy that is left over. If conception is eluding you, stress is the most likely culprit. Indeed, long-term stress can even cause medical problems that require medical solutions. Regular yoga practice is a simple preventative measure and can also be a cure. It increases your energy supply and channels it to all the body's systems to keep them in balance so that you become fit and relaxed, living each moment to the full.

what your body language tells you

The way you sit, stand and move can reveal a lot about your state of mind, health and emotional well-being at any time. If most of your energy is tied up either in your mind (your work, for example), in your emotions (say, problems that may be weighing on your mind) or in your hectic lifestyle, your body becomes depleted. There just may not be enough energy left over to work your reproductive system properly. It can be as simple as that. This stress can be reflected in your body language – legs tightly crossed, upper spine hunched over, or arms crossed over your chest.

"This state, in which the senses are steady and at rest, is known as yoga, the state of union."

Katha Upanishad VI 9

The yogic answer to stress is to rebalance your nervous and endocrine systems so that all functions are enhanced. Use yoga to stretch, strengthen, open and relax. This releases locked-up energy, and so eases conception, pregnancy and birth.

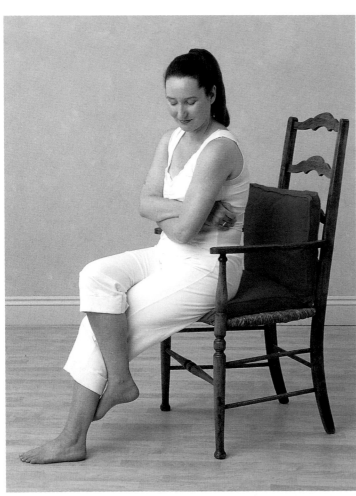

△ The "uptight" body language here says it all. This posture displays feelings of fear and vulnerability. The arms and legs form a shield across the trunk, blocking the flow of energy. The chest and abdomen are closed, so that breathing is restricted and energy to the pelvic area is blocked.

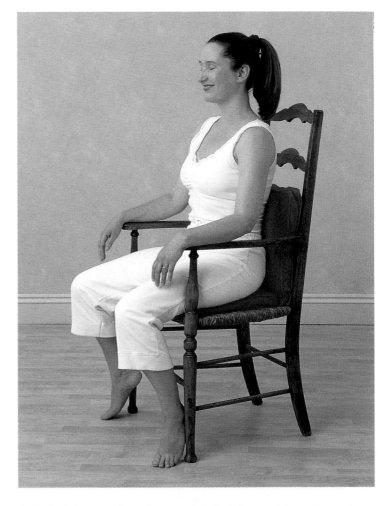

△ The body language here shows a relaxed mind, peaceful emotions and an erect, vibrant spine. The shoulders, neck, hips and pelvis are relaxed so that energy can flow freely throughout the body.

breath is the key

The respiratory and cardiovascular systems bring oxygen (the prime source of energy) into the body from the outside air and circulate it to every cell. Good breathing habits, therefore, increase the total supply of energy available for the body's systems to use. The diaphragm is the large muscle that separates the abdomen from the chest cavity. It is the chief breathing muscle. If its movement is restricted through poor posture it cannot pump enough air into the lungs and so not enough oxygen is available to the body. Shallow breathing, which does not draw in enough oxygen, is one of the main causes of feeling below par. Deep breathing (using the diaphragm fully) is instantly energizing.

As you breathe in, the diaphragm contracts strongly downwards, massaging and energizing the abdominal organs and increasing lung capacity so that air rushes in, through the nose, from outside. The diaphragm springs back up again as you breathe out, releasing the abdominal pressure and decreasing the lung capacity so that air is forced out through the nose. This contraction and release reflects the whole momentum of yoga – activity followed by rest, followed by activity, in a continuous, balanced cycle. Practised with awareness, deep breathing reconnects us with this rhythm of life and helps us to learn how to relax deeply between all bouts of activity. It also helps to create a calm strength.

1 Tuning in to your breath

A deep breath in recharges both body and mind. A deep breath out releases muscular tension, chemical waste products and tired, strained feelings. Mentally, take your breath in to the very base of your spine. Taking time to practise breathing slowly, deeply and fully induces calm, positive feelings.

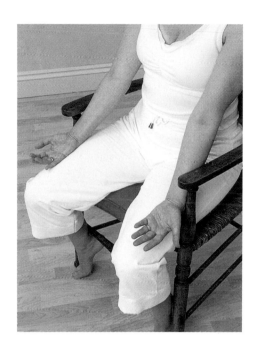

◁ Sit at the back of a firm chair with spine erect, knees apart and feet on the floor. Rest your hands with palms up in an open, receptive gesture. This position opens the trunk, so the diaphragm can move freely. Take several deep breaths with awareness of what is happening to your body as you breathe. Repeat the exercise frequently.

CAUTION
Deep breathing is strenuous, especially if it is new to you. Stop at once if you feel tired, breathless or light-headed. Rest for a while before starting again. Very gradually build up the number of deep breaths you take at any one time.

2 Flexibility in the pelvis

The reproductive system lies within the lower part of the abdomen and is protected by the bony pelvic girdle. This area needs to be open and relaxed so that energy can circulate freely through the reproductive system and conception is unhindered. Regular movement of the pelvis brings energy, flexibility and strength to this area.

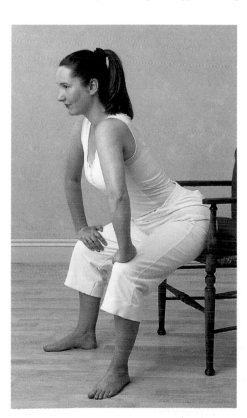

◁ **1** Sit on the edge of a sturdy chair with feet apart and set firmly on the floor. Place your hands on your thighs above your knees, with fingers turned in and elbows turned out. Lean forward, bend your elbows and take your upper body weight on your thighs. This frees the pelvis – think of it as a bowl and tip it forward at the front "rim" (the pubic bone) and up at the back "rim" (where the sacrum joins the spine).

▷ **2** Open the front of the body by spreading your arms with palms up, lifting your chest and tucking your pelvis under so that the front pelvic "rim" rises and the back "rim" is lowered. This movement stretches the spine and releases tension. It also tightens the lower abdominal muscles that hold the pelvis in place. Repeat these two movements several times and practise frequently in order to increase mobility in the pelvic area.

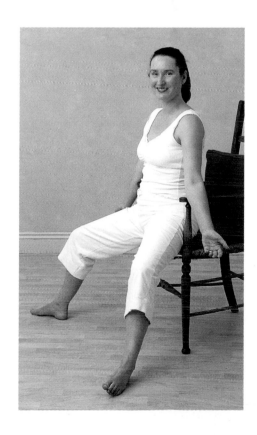

breath awareness

healthy conception

As well as energizing the body, our breathing has a profound influence on the nervous system. Fast or shallow breathing makes us feel anxious and stressed, whereas slow, deep breathing immediately relaxes us. If you are to practise active relaxation, you need to be aware of your breathing patterns, so that you can use your breath to consciously reduce stress and promote well-being. Note that the awareness of exhalation comes first in yoga, avoiding any forceful inhalation.

3 Deepening the breath

Sit upright on a sturdy chair, with your feet apart and planted firmly on the floor. Feel your breathing muscles working by placing your hands on your ribs, then lower chest, then abdomen. The lower you can take the breathing movement the more energized and relaxed you will feel, and the more efficiently your abdominal organs (digestive and reproductive) can function. In yoga you should always breathe in and out through the nose unless instructed otherwise.

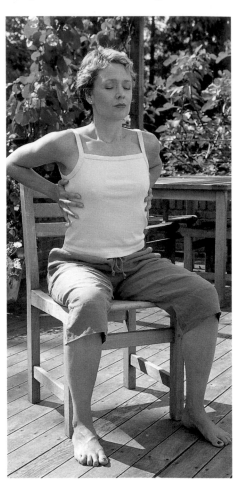
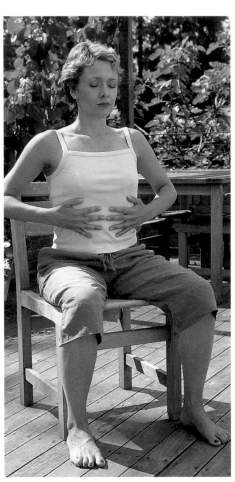
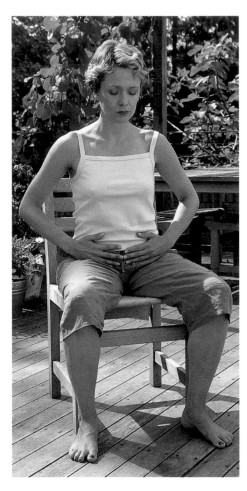

△ **1** Bring your elbows back to open your chest, and place your hands on the sides of your ribs with fingers pointing forward. Breathe in deeply, expanding your ribcage against your hands. Breathe out, keeping the lift and openness in the chest. Be careful not to collapse, even though your ribcage contracts a little. Repeat several times.

△ **2** Still with elbows wide and chest open, bring your hands forward with fingers pointing towards each other and little fingers against your lowest ribs. As you breathe in feel your lower ribs expanding outwards and your diaphragm contracting downwards against your abdominal organs. As you breathe out feel the ribs relaxing inwards and the diaphragm relaxing upwards. Repeat several times. If you blow the air out forcibly through your mouth you will also feel the corset muscles around your waist contracting sharply.

△ **3** Now move your hands below the navel to feel the effect of deep breathing on the abdominal organs. As you breathe in, contracting the diaphragm, the downward pressure massages and flushes away stale blood from these organs. As you breathe out this pressure is released and fresh new blood rushes in, bringing a new supply of oxygen and nutrients. Feel the movements of your breathing reaching right down through the abdomen and pelvis to the muscular pelvic floor. Repeat a few times, keeping neck and shoulders relaxed, and then rest.

4 Stretch, bend and relax

This exercise sets the pattern for all your yoga practice – alternating active movements with a pause to relax. If you can arrange your daily life to the same natural rhythm you will find that you can undo stress before it has a chance to build up. Either sitting or standing you can rid the lungs of stale air, open the chest and massage the abdominal organs.

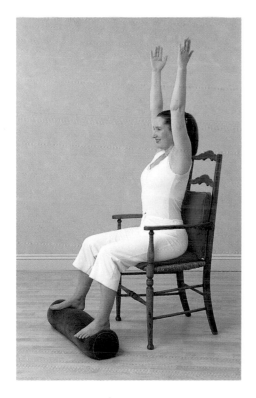

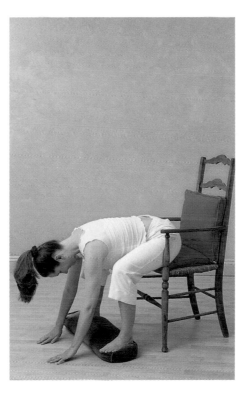

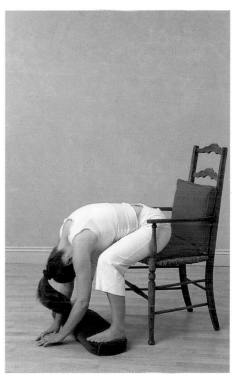

△**1** Make sure that you are seated comfortably and use a firm bolster or similar as a foot support. As you breathe in raise both straight arms above your head.

△ **2** As you breathe out fold forward like a rag doll, dropping your head between your knees and hands loosely to the floor.

△ **3** Breathing naturally, relax your neck and shoulders to ease out any tension. Repeat this exercise several times.

5 Lengthening the outbreath

The breath out relaxes the nervous system, whereas the breath in is energizing. First, sigh or yawn to release tension. Always remember to make the breath out last a little longer than the breath in. An enjoyable way to lengthen the breath out is by using the voice. A lower pitch usually resonates better than a higher one and is more relaxing.

▷ With spine erect and chest open, breathe in deeply and let the air out slowly as you chant "A...E...I...O...U...".

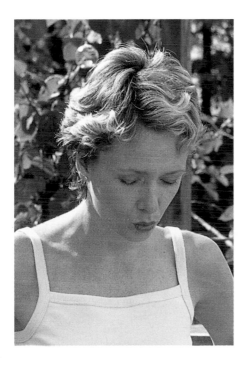

6 Alternate nostril breathing

This breathing exercise is a classical yoga practice. It is remarkable for soothing the nervous system and balancing our extrovert and introvert tendencies – calming us when we are anxious or overexcited and lifting our spirits when we are tired or depressed. Ideally, it should be practised for a few minutes each day.

▷ Sit with spine erect and chest open. Place the right hand in front of the face, with the index and middle finger resting lightly on the centre of the forehead, the thumb in position to close the right nostril, and the ring finger in position to close the left nostril. Now concentrate and follow these steps:
• Close the right nostril with the thumb and breathe in through the left nostril.
• Close the left nostril and open the right.
• Breathe out through the right nostril.
• Breathe in through the right nostril.
• Close the right nostril and open the left. Breathe out through the left nostril.

This is one round. Repeat, gradually building up the number of rounds over a few weeks.

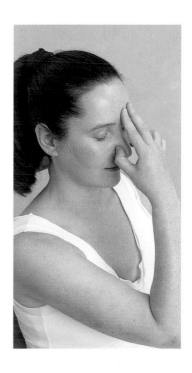

Yoga poses to release tension

healthy conception

For many people, tension seems to settle in the pelvic region, causing stiffness in the hips, pain in the lower back, and general congestion and an uptight feeling in the lower abdominal area. Yoga stretches relieve all these conditions and allow energy to circulate freely once more. They also work on the whole body, so remember to keep the spine extended and the chest open in all these exercises.

CAUTION
Make haste slowly. Widen your legs and stretch to the side and forwards only as far as you comfortably can. Locked-in tension impedes movement and should never be fought against. As you release the tension through yoga movements, you will find it easier to move much further and to relax more deeply into the positions. All yoga stretching should be performed with active relaxation and not force or effort.

7 Seated looseners

Let your partner encourage and help you. It is fun and relaxing for both of you. The closeness of trying to conceive can permeate all aspects of your life together.

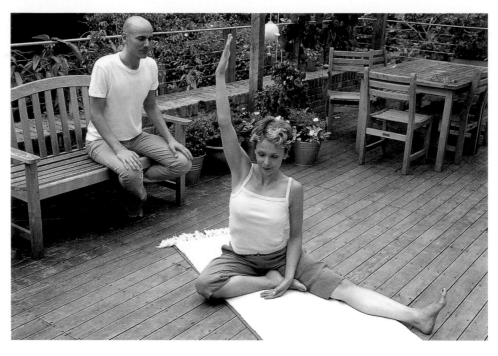

△ **1** Sit on the floor (on a yoga mat or piece of non-slip carpet) with legs extended and feet comfortably far apart. Bend your right knee and bring your foot to rest against your left inner thigh, with your heel as close to the pubic bone as possible. Flex your left ankle and straighten your left knee. Raise your right arm overhead and stretch up through your right side, breathing in.

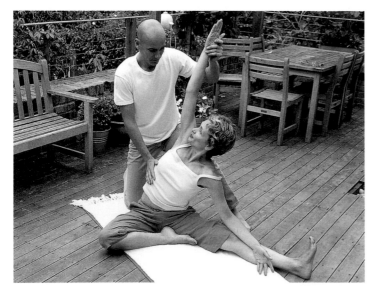

△ **2** Breathe out as you lean to the left over your left leg, with your left arm sliding gently along your leg and your right arm stretching up. Breathe in as you sit up, lowering your right arm.

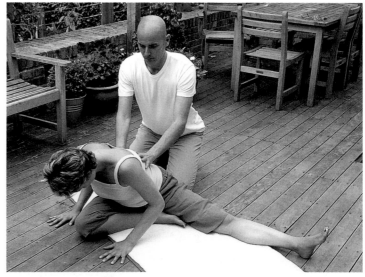

△ **3** Breathe out as you bend to the right, walking your hands along the floor each side of your bent right leg. Keep the left ankle flexed and stretch right through your left side as you bend over your right leg. Breathe in as you sit up straight. Repeat these movements a few times on the same side. Then breathe naturally as you change legs and repeat the movements with the left knee bent.

8 Kneeling looseners

Loosening movements can also be performed using a sofa or bench for leverage, so that you can get a strong twist in the upper body while keeping your spine extended and erect, and hips in position.

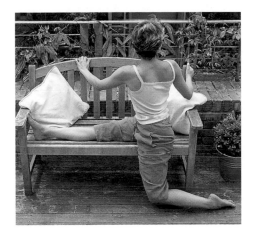

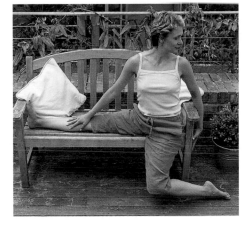

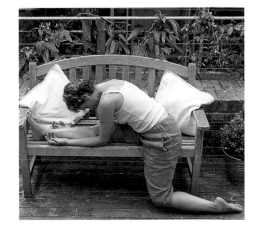

△1 Kneel with your right side against the bench, then raise your right leg and place it along the bench seat. Keep your ankle flexed. Hold the back of the bench and breathe in. As you breathe out, pull your upper body around to the right, keeping your spine erect and chest open. Breathe in again to face forward.

△ 2 Place your right hand against your inner right leg and use the arm of the bench to lever your upper body round to the left as you breathe out. Breathe in to face forward again.

△3 Breathe out to lean forward and slide your upturned hands alongside your straight right leg. Breathe in as you sit up straight. Repeat these movements a few times on the same side, then turn around and repeat to stretch the other side.

9 Happy womb poses

It is important to focus your attention in the lower abdomen and to create space there in order to bring more energy to the reproductive system. Sit on the floor or a chair and open your hips, with your knees wide apart, as often as possible. You can sit comfortably on the floor to read, talk on the phone, watch TV and do most of those things you normally do sitting in a chair – only in a chair the pelvic area is apt to be constricted, especially if you cross your legs.

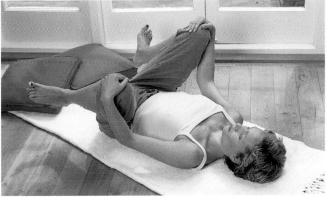

◁ 1 Lie on your back, bend your knees and hold one knee in each hand. Keeping your chin tucked down and your waist against the floor (using the abdominal muscles), rotate your knees outwards with your hands, relaxing and opening the hip joints. Circle the knees out and in again for a few moments, several times a day.

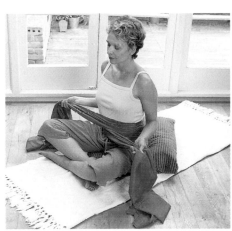

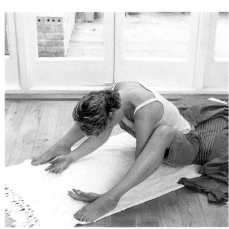

△ 2 Sit upright with your legs loosely crossed and a scarf around your middle, crossed over at the abdomen. As you breathe out pull the scarf ends loosely to create pressure. Breathe in deeply against this pressure to open the scarf and bring the breathing movements down into the lower abdomen and pelvic floor. Continue for several minutes.

△ 3 Sit with your knees bent and your feet apart and flat on the floor. Now bring your palms together with bent elbows. Keeping your chest open, gently press your elbows against your inner thighs for a few moments to open the hip joints. Breathe slowly and deeply.

△ 4 Remaining seated, lean forward and place your hands on the floor with palms upwards. Gently press your knees apart with your upper arms. Breathe deeply, lengthening the out-breath for as long as you can.

Nearly effortless stretches

Physical movement increases blood flow, and therefore the supply of oxygen, to the part of the body that is being moved – bringing new fuel (and thus energy) to the cellular structures. This blood flow also removes accumulated waste products, which can cause harmful imbalances if allowed to build up.

Awareness focused on any part of the body also brings vital energy to that part, since energy follows thought. The following exercises are done lying down because this allows maximum relaxation of the nervous system.

10 Pelvic movements with focused awareness

These relaxing movements encourage increased awareness, blood flow and flexibility in the pelvic area. Feel that you are opening up to new healing energy and letting go of any tension there.

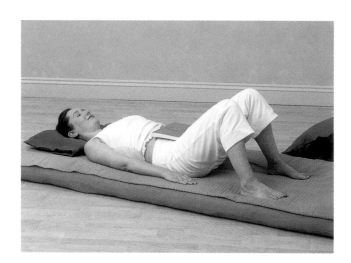

◁ **1** Lie on your back, with a large book and three cushions beside you. Place one cushion under your head and tuck your chin in to lengthen the back of your neck. Bend your knees and plant your feet hip-width apart on the floor. Place the book on your lower abdomen, so that it is evenly balanced upon the hip bones and the pubic bone, then stretch your arms alongside your body with the palms down to support you.

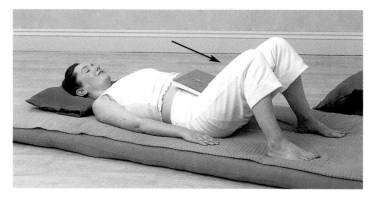

△ **2** As you breathe in press on your hands and arch your lower back as much as you can, so that the navel and hip bones rise and the front "rim" of your pelvis (and the book) is tipped towards your feet.

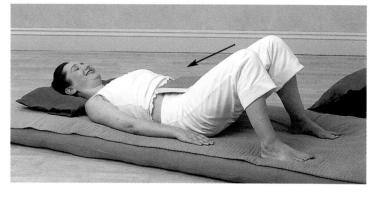

△ **3** As you breathe out pull the navel against the spine and press on your hands to lift the coccyx just off the floor, so that the pelvic front "rim" (and the book) is now tipped backward, towards your head. Keep your waist against the floor and move the lower spine only. Repeat steps 1–3 several times.

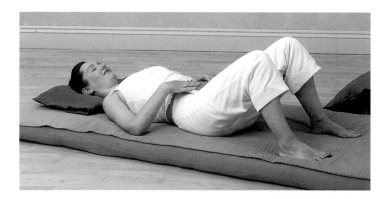

△ **4** Now place your hands, in a relaxed pose, on top of the book and breathe deeply. Feel the movements of the book over the pelvic area as you breathe in and out slowly for several minutes.

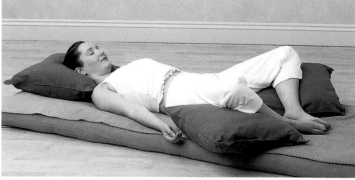

△ **5** Remove the book and bring the soles of your feet together so that your knees fall outward. Support them with the remaining two cushions. Place your hands, palms up, beside you in a gesture of openness and complete surrender. Relax for several minutes.

11 Improving flexibility and muscle tone

Here are three simple exercises to improve flexibility in the spine and hips and to strengthen the abdominal muscles. They may seem strenuous to begin with, but strength and flexibility will improve rapidly with practice. Relax afterwards and feel the effects of the exercises on your muscles and your breath. Keep your coccyx on the floor throughout.

▷ **1** Lie on your back with a cushion under your head and your arms, palms down, alongside the body to support you. Bend your right leg, keeping your left leg stretched with the ankle flexed. Make large cycling circles with your right leg until you feel tired. Then rest with both legs stretched out and become aware of the muscles you have been working in the right side of the lower abdomen. Repeat the same number of circles with your left leg, and then rest again.

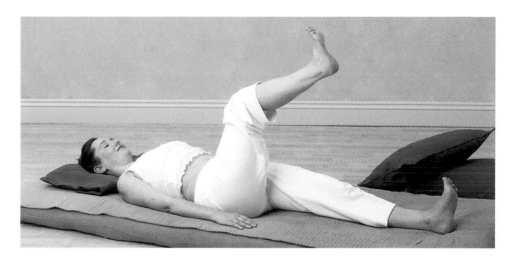

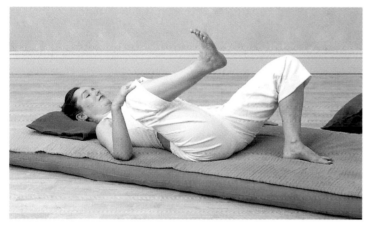

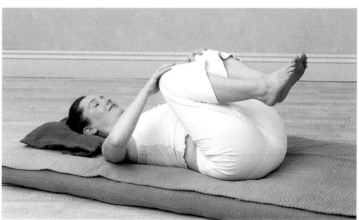

△ **2** With your left knee bent and left foot planted firmly on the floor, take hold of your right knee and move the right leg in circles from the hip. This releases tightness in the groin and hip joint. Rest, then repeat the movements on the other side.

△ **3** Now work with both knees and the breath. Breathe in as you take the knees out to the sides. Breathe out as you pull your knees close to your chest to stretch your lower back. Repeat several times then rest.

12 Lying twist

This powerful but simple twisting exercise opens up and relaxes both the shoulders and the hips. This in turn helps to make the entire spine more flexible, creating space between the vertebrae.

▷ Lie down, raise your arms, bent at the elbows, and place them on the floor above or beside your head. This position opens and lifts the chest. Bend your knees and place your feet together on the floor. Breathe in. As you breathe out lower both knees to the right, ensuring that you keep them together. The aim is to place your right knee on the floor without letting your left elbow leave the floor, but only take it as far as feels comfortable. As you breathe in raise your knees to the centre, still keeping them pressed together. As you breathe out lower them to the left and raise them again as you breathe in. Repeat until tired, then relax for several minutes.

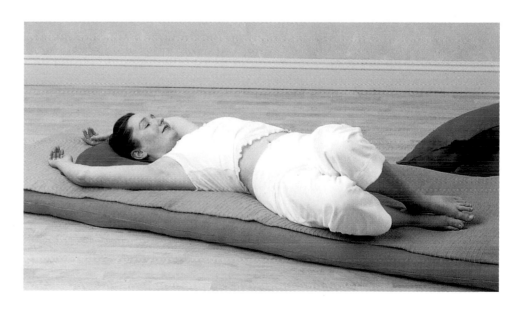

Sharing energy with your partner

Do you lack quality time with your partner? It may be that you are both so busy that you hardly ever have time simply to enjoy each other's company. Yogic stretching, relaxing and unwinding together may be all that is needed to make your womb, and his sperm, more "conception friendly".

Nature often works on a subliminal level and an openness and emotional intimacy with each other can increase the likelihood of conception. Remember too, that prolonged stress can adversely affect the reproductive systems of both sexes, and that

yoga gradually dissolves the effects of past stress and also helps to prevent new stress from building up.

Couples are very often disappointed if conception does not occur exactly when they are ready for it, especially as preparing for a baby involves great shifts in outlook and investments of energy. Yoga helps to deepen harmony and acceptance between hopeful parents at this difficult stage.

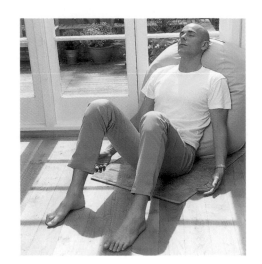

▷ **Teach your partner the joys of yoga relaxation. Stress affects his reproductive capabilities too.**

13 Moving energy into your reproductive system

Every single message passing along your nervous system between the brain and the body has to go through the neck. It is hardly surprising that the neck and shoulders often get tense and energy-congested. Massage releases this congestion and allows energy to move freely around the body once again.

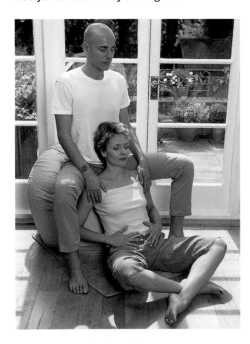

△ Encourage your partner to massage your neck and shoulders to restore energy flow while you place your hands on your abdomen and focus on "charging" your ovaries with deep breathing. Then change places so that you can massage his neck and shoulders.

14 Synchronizing your energies

When both partners are relaxed, synchronized and emotionally ready for conception – "two hearts beating as one" – a favourable energy field will help conception to take place.

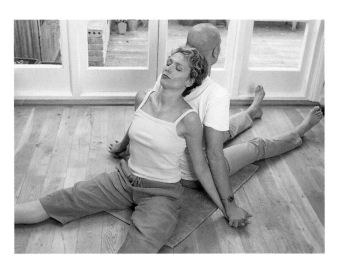

◁ **1** Sit back to back so that the flow of energy in your spines can synchronize, bringing you closer together on an energy level. You will find that your breathing also synchronizes as you relax into each other and become much more intimate.

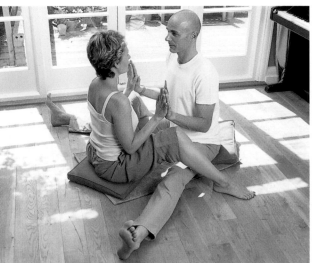

◁ **2** To become even closer, sit facing each other with spines straight. Place your legs over your partner's legs, snuggle up, place your palms against his and gaze into each other's eyes. Your energies will synchronize and pass from one to the other through your eyes and your joined palms.

A sample practice for promoting conception

1
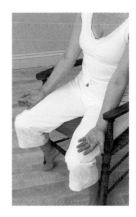
▷ **Tuning in to
your breath (1)**

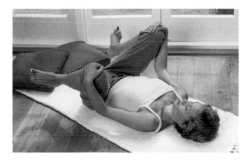
2 △ **Happy womb pose (9)**

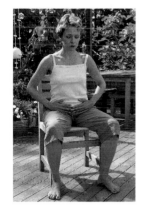
3 ◁ **Deepening
the breath (3)**

4
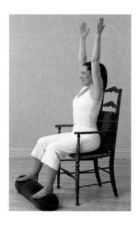
◁ **Stretch, bend
and relax (4)**

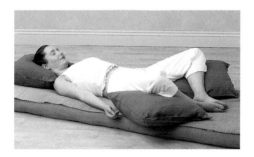
5 △ **Pelvic movements with focused
awareness (10)**

6
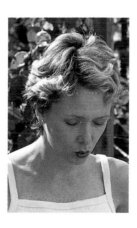
▷ **Lengthening the
outbreath (5)**

Questions and answers

• **Roughly how long should we try to conceive before consulting
medical experts?**

If you have been taking oral contraceptives for years and then
stop in order to conceive, your reproductive system may take up
to a year to re-establish its natural rhythm. If you and your
partner have stressful jobs you may need to take steps to change
your lifestyles so that you can both reduce your stress levels.
Yoga practice speeds up the rate at which you de-stress. Medical
intervention may ultimately be needed but remember that
medical procedures are in themselves stressful – so do what you
can to help yourselves first. Remember also that there is no
definite answer – everyone is different.

• **We have had all the medical tests recommended to us and there is
nothing wrong with either of us. What can we do now?**

If both of you have undergone tests that have revealed nothing,
there may be simple reasons why you have not conceived yet.
The most common reason is simply that it can take a long time
– always far too long when you are waiting eagerly. Highly
subtle psychological and physiological changes can make a
difference here. For example, the slight shifts in pH levels – in
both you and your partner – that can arise from continued yoga
and relaxation practices, could help to lead you further down
the road to conception.

• **What are the chances of success with IVF procedures?**

Only medical experts can advise you in your particular case.
IVF procedures are increasingly successful.

• **I just can't relax. What am I doing wrong?**

Getting uptight about relaxing in order to conceive! It is better
to learn to relax in order to reduce the stress in your life. This
then creates an atmosphere where conception becomes more
likely. Go on holiday with your partner and practise yoga
together away from your daily routine. Make plans to simplify
your lives when you get home so that you can enjoy more
quality time together. Make yoga part of your life and use your
positive affirmations each day. Most importantly, affirm your
blessings with regard to what you already have in life.

• **I have a specific medical problem (such as having just one ovary) that
makes conception difficult.**

A positive attitude is a great help in overcoming all kinds of
obstacles, but we also have to cultivate an open, accepting
disposition that will enable us to embrace our life equally well if
conception remains elusive. Seek expert medical help and keep
as healthy and relaxed as possible. Use regular yogic exercise,
breathing, relaxation and meditation practices to keep all the
systems of your body running as smoothly as possible.

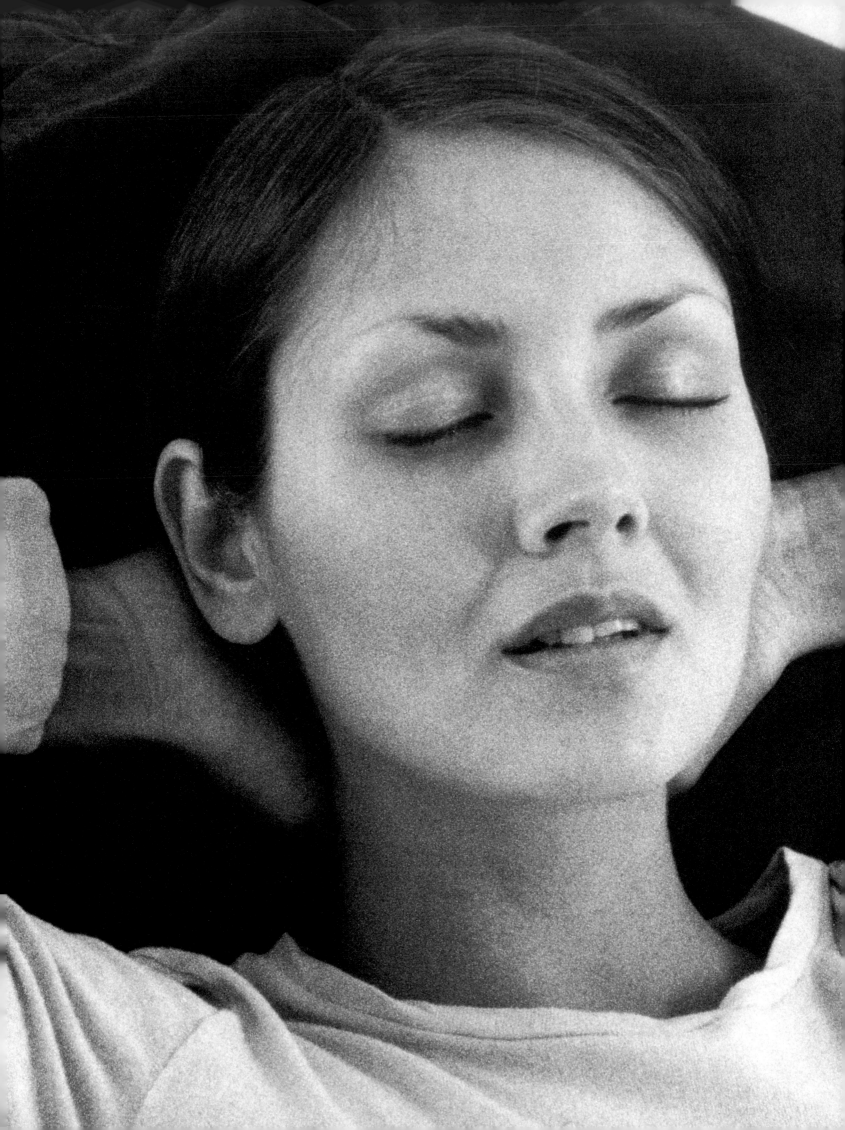

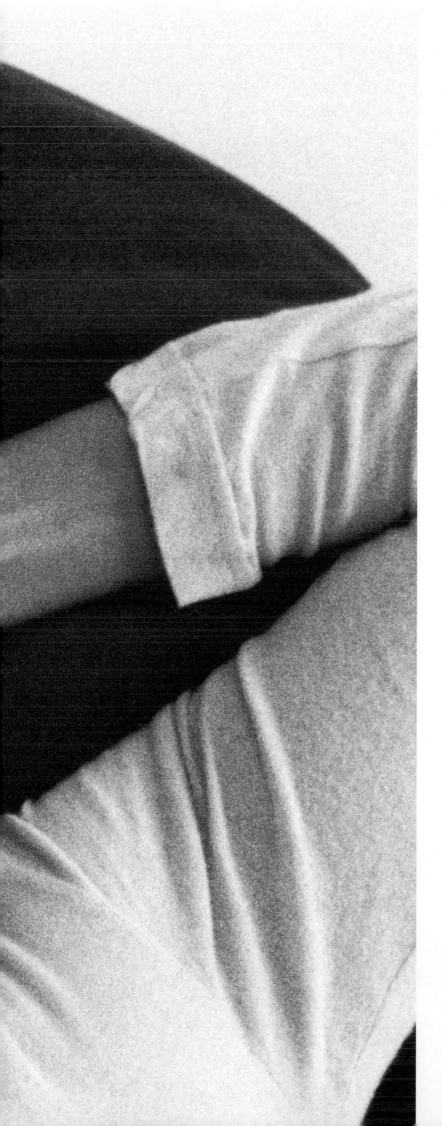

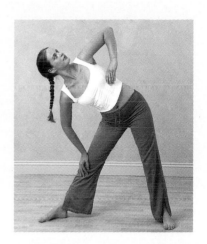

1–14
weeks

Congratulations on becoming pregnant!
Right from the moment of conception,
Nature's first priority is the welfare of the
fetus growing in the womb. Your own
needs take second place now. While your
body is adjusting to this totally new
situation – which can take up to 14 weeks
– your hormonal balance is fragile, so it is
important to conserve your energy and to
respond to your body's needs rather than
trying to ignore them.

Make space in your life for your pregnancy

No doubt you already realize that you will have to re-arrange your priorities once your baby is born. However, the best time to start is right now. Making a baby requires a lot of energy, but our energy is limited, especially if we lead busy lives. That energy must come from somewhere and therefore, since Nature ensures that your baby comes first and gets all it needs to develop, it is vital that you conserve and boost your own energy levels. Yoga conserves energy by reducing stress through deep relaxation and boosts it by increasing your oxygen uptake through yogic deep breathing and movement.

get the yoga habit now

Yoga will stand you in good stead right through your pregnancy, after your baby is born and for the rest of your life. You will soon be hooked on the sense of well-being that it brings. Your daily session can be quite short, as long as it is regular, and many yoga techniques can be incorporated into daily life. As you become more aware of your posture, emotions, thoughts and attitudes, you will want to adjust them, whatever you happen to be doing and wherever you are.

learn to nurture yourself

Many women feel that they should hide their feelings, ignore their needs, always appear strong and independent and keep going, no matter what. But you must learn to stop, relax and nurture yourself. Only when you know what it feels like to be loved will you have the capacity to nurture the life in your womb and care for a tiny baby. Practise being vulnerable and learn to ask for help and support from your loved ones.

CAUTION
Whether or not you have practised yoga before, keep it very easy and simple for the first 14 weeks of your pregnancy. Focus on breathing and relaxation rather than movement.

15 Feet up the wall sequence

This relaxing sequence rests tired legs and lower back, while stretching the muscles in the groin and preparing the muscles of the pelvic floor. Meanwhile, practise slow, deep breathing with awareness.

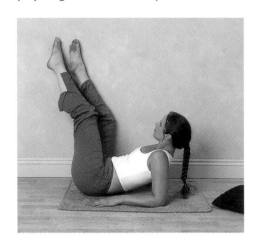

△1 Sit with the legs along a wall. It is best to bend the inner knee, lean back on the hands and then forearms, and swivel your bottom round before raising the legs.

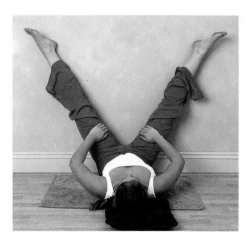

△ 2 Swivel your upper body round and straighten your legs against the wall – buttocks and legs should touch the wall. Place a cushion under your head.

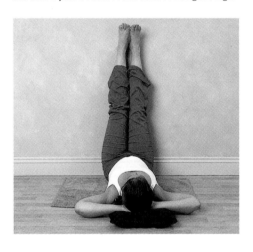

△ 3 Place your hands under your head with elbows on the floor, to open up your chest. Breathe deeply for a few moments.

△ 4 Take your legs comfortably apart to release tightness in the pelvis and groin. Gently massage the inner thighs while breathing deeply.

◁ 5 Bend your knees and slide the soles of your feet down the wall, a comfortable width apart. Place your hands over your lower abdomen and become aware of your pelvic floor muscles. Draw in the muscles as you breathe in, and release the tension gently as you breathe out. Repeat several times.

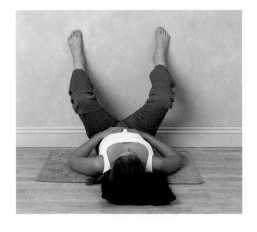

16 Lying down stretches

A similar exercise helps to relax the pelvic region for conception but it is just as effective here, where the point of focus is the lower back. The lumbar region of the spine, the sacrum and the coccyx should all relax against the floor – quite easy when the knees are bent and pulled gently toward the chest. If muscular tension prevents the lower spine from softening in this position, take long deep breaths out to relax more fully. The gentle movements will further ease your lower back and remove any stiffness or soreness.

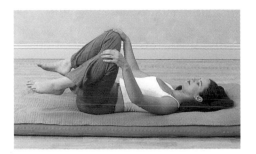

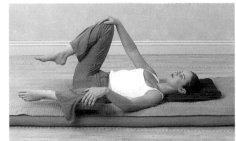

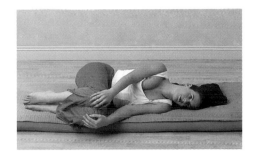

△ **1** Lie on your back with your spine long and chin down. Keeping your coccyx on the floor, take one bent knee in each hand. Bring your knees toward your chest then gently circle them out to the sides to massage your lower back against the floor. This is a great way to release backache. Repeat several times.

△ **2** Gently bring one knee toward the floor. As far as possible, make sure that both shoulders remain relaxed and your back stays flat against the floor. Keep your neck relaxed and breathe deeply.

△ **3** Breathe out as you roll on to one side, bringing your knees together. Relax in this position and breathe deeply. Breathe in to roll on to your back, raising first one knee and then the other, or both together if you can. Repeat on the other side.

17 The bridge pose

This pose strengthens the leg muscles, especially the inner thighs, which helps you to support the extra weight of your baby as the pregnancy progresses. The Bridge Pose also stretches the muscles around the groin area, opens the chest and frees the diaphragm for deeper breathing. Alternate this exercise with the previous one so that you both relax and strengthen the lower spine and abdominal muscles. This will bring awareness and energy to the whole area.

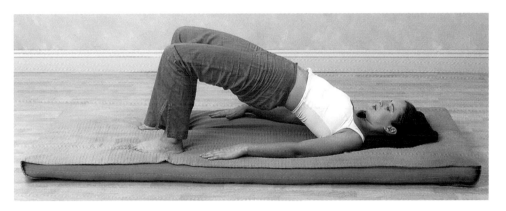

△ Place your feet flat on the floor near your buttocks, about hip-width apart. Stretch your arms alongside your body, palms down, for support. Breathe in and raise your pelvis off the floor. Breathe deeply a few times in this position. Slowly lower your buttocks to the floor on a long breath out. Repeat several times.

18 Deep relaxation with focused breathing

Leave enough time so that you can end every yoga session with deep relaxation. It quickly dissolves any stress that may have built up, removing muscular tension and congestion and bringing new energy to all the body's systems.

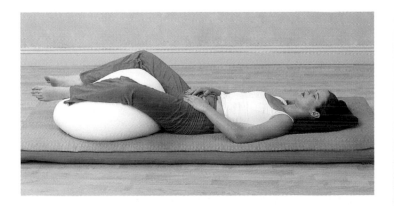

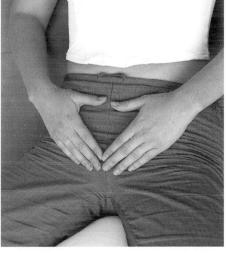

◁ **2** Place your palms over your lower abdomen, thumbs touching. Breathe deeply, and feel which is the best hand position to soothe you and bring nourishment to your baby. Close your eyes and relax.

△ **1** Lie on your back with your spine long and chin down. Drape your legs over a beanbag or a pile of cushions, with knees bent out to the sides. Bring your heels close together and relax your feet.

A strong, supple spine supports your baby

Good posture is especially important during pregnancy for the following reasons.

- It holds your womb, in which your baby lies, in its correct position in the lower abdomen. This makes your pregnancy a far more comfortable experience for both of you.
- It relieves backache and can avoid its onset.
- It creates more space in the chest and abdominal areas, which become increasingly crowded by the presence of the growing baby.

- It improves breathing, and therefore your energy levels, because it gives the diaphragm more room to move.
- It improves digestion, which cannot function properly if there is compression in the abdomen.
- It prevents congestion in the circulatory system to the womb, upon which your baby depends for all its nourishment.
- It streamlines your figure, however large or small the bump.

- It makes you feel great. Standing and walking tall express a positive outlook, whereas the general compression and congestion that result from poor posture can make your energy stagnate and your mood depressed.

Although changes to your figure may be hard to detect in the early days, especially in your first pregnancy, it is important to concentrate on your posture from the start, before any bad habits are established.

19 Dog pose

This pose lengthens the spine and increases spinal awareness, as well as strengthening the muscles in the upper back, arms and hands. It also improves circulation and releases tension across the shoulders, and in the neck and face. Below are three variations on the Dog Pose. Try them all out and see which one suits you best.

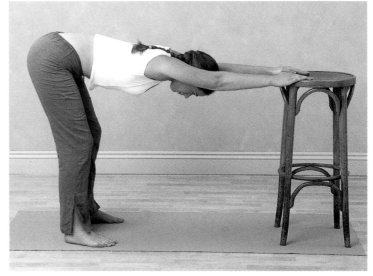

▷ **Pose 1** Hold on to a table, stool or radiator and step away from it until your spine and arms are stretched and horizontal to the floor, and your feet are hip-width apart. It helps initially if someone checks that your back is flat. Keep your head and neck horizontal, so that your ears are in line with your arms. Breathe deeply and bend your knees slightly if this helps you stretch further.

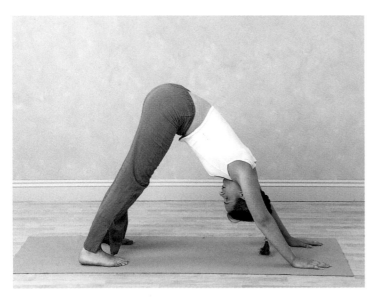

△ **Pose 2** Make a right angle by walking your hands forward (shoulder-width apart) with knees bent. Straighten your legs (feet hip-width apart) on a breath out, bringing your heels to the floor if you can. As you breathe in stretch through the spine and arms. Hold the pose for a few breaths, breathing deeply.

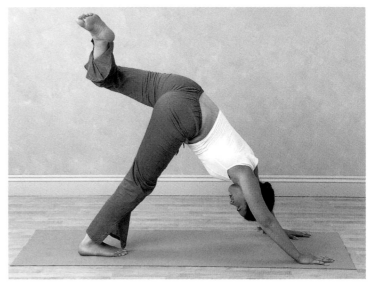

△ **Pose 3** From the position shown in Pose 2, balance on one leg and raise the other. Keep the knee of the leg that is on the floor bent. Push down into your arms and hands. Now change legs to repeat on the other side.

20 Alignment of the spine

Your posture can be improved simply by becoming aware and straightening up whenever you notice that you are drooping. The back of the body, being bonier than the front, has less sensation (fewer nerve endings), so it is quite difficult to be aware of the position of your spine. It helps to stand or sit against a surface such as a wall, so you can feel whether your muscles are holding your spine firmly upright or are slack. With practice, both awareness and posture will improve as you locate and strengthen the relevant muscles.

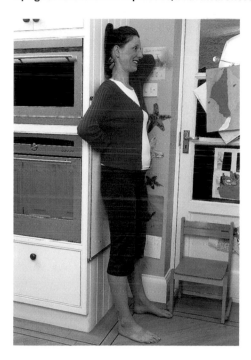

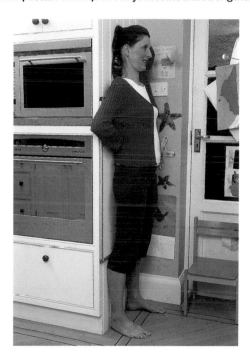

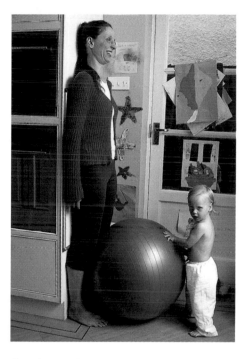

△ **1** Stand with feet a short distance from the wall and hands behind your waist. Press against the wall with head, shoulders, waist and buttocks. Lengthen your neck, lowering your chin. Breathe in and stand as tall as you can. Hold this stretch and contact with the wall as you breathe out. Repeat a few times.

△ **2** Now bring your heels and calves against the wall and repeat the same stretch up as you breathe in, maintaining contact with the wall as you breathe out. Repeat.

△ **3** Bring your hands to your sides and press your waist against the wall as you stretch up, breathing in. Maintain contact with the wall as you breathe out. Repeat.

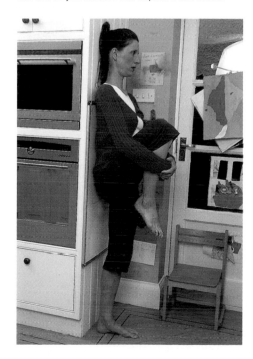

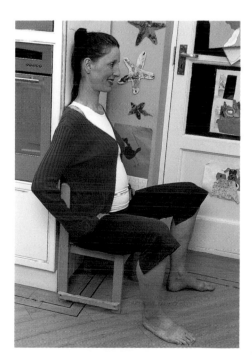

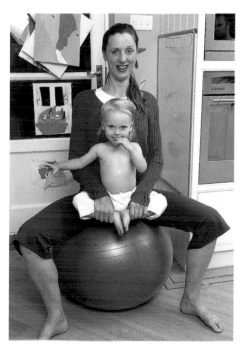

△ **4** Bend one knee and clasp both hands around your shin. Draw your thigh close to your chest as you breathe out, balancing on your straight leg. Release the pull on your shin as you breathe in and stretch up, maintaining contact with the wall. Repeat.

△ **5** Sit on a low stool with knees apart and feet firmly planted on the floor. Maintain contact with the wall with your head, shoulders, waist and buttocks as you breathe in and stretch up, then breathe out and hold the upward stretch.

△ **6** Once you have found and strengthened your spinal muscles, practise lifting up through your spine whenever you are standing or sitting.

Easy standing poses

Now that you have learnt how to keep your spine aligned, and know how good that feels, you can maintain the alignment as you move gracefully through these sequences. They develop strength and suppleness, helping you to protect and nourish your growing baby as well as yourself. They also help to keep your feet firmly on the ground and remain steady as your body changes.

21 Grounding

The joints and muscles around your hips, legs and feet take the weight of your whole body, and the muscles of the pelvis and pelvic floor carry the weight of your upper body and trunk. These important muscle groups can be strengthened and toned by the following grounding exercise, which allows your weight to pass smoothly through your legs and feet into the ground beneath you. It becomes ever more important to work with gravity rather than against it as your baby becomes heavier.

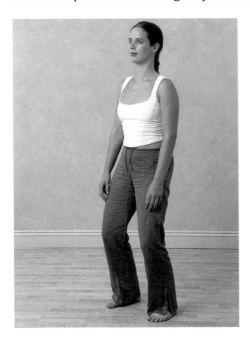

△ **1** Stand with your feet apart and loosely bend your knees, making sure you maintain your upright posture through the spine.

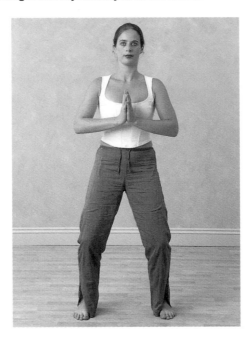

△ **2** Bring your hands into Namaste, the prayer position, and press your palms firmly together with elbows out to the sides.

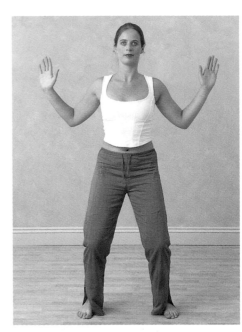

△ **3** Spread your hands wide, so that you keep your elbows bent and open up your chest area, all the time breathing in deeply.

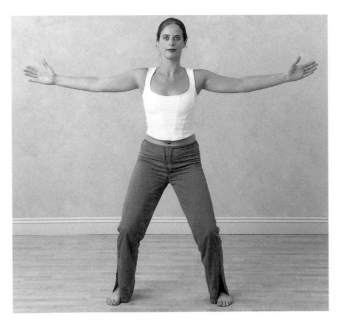

◁ **4** Stretch your arms out to the sides and lower them, breathing out. Repeat steps 1 to 4 several times.

▷ **5** For a stronger version of this exercise, place one foot on a low chair and bend the other knee. Change legs after a few breaths and repeat with the other foot on the chair.

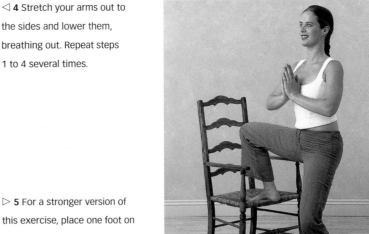

22 Standing stretches

By stretching up from the hips and through the waist, these stretches create space for the diaphragm to contract downwards to a greater extent, so that you breathe more deeply. Twist and sway rhythmically as if you are dancing.

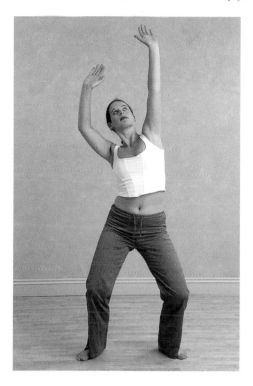

◁ **1** Stand with knees loosely bent and stretch your arms overhead, first one side and then the other. Feel your ribs and waist opening and releasing.

▷ **2** Now bring your arms out at shoulder level and swing round from the waist, first to one side and then the other, without changing your leg or arm position. Repeat both movements.

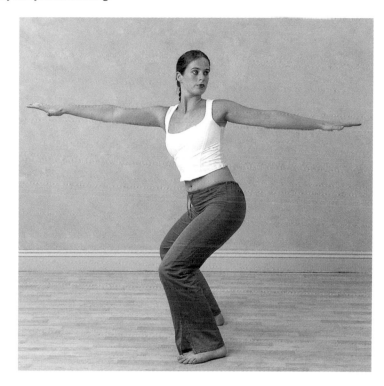

23 Adapted easy triangle sequence

This sequence works out your oblique abdominal muscles and your lumbar spine. Strong obliques help to prevent backache, hold your developing baby firmly and trim your figure.

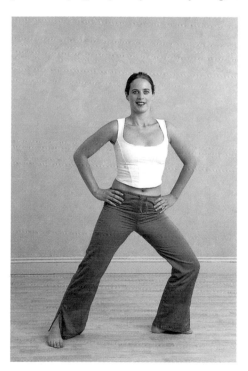

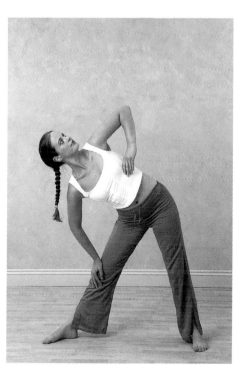

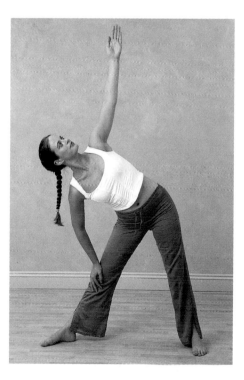

△ **1** Stand tall with feet wide and knees well bent. Place your hands on your hips and sway from side to side, tipping your pelvis up to the right as you sway to the right and up to the left as you sway to the left in a rhythmical movement. Keep your spine erect, coccyx tucked under and chest lifted. Repeat the sequence several times to loosen the hips and pelvis.

△ **2** Bend to your right side without tipping forward. Place your right hand along your leg and bring your left elbow back to open the left side of the waist and chest as you look upwards.

△ **3** Now stretch your left arm right up and back to open the left side of your body. Repeat the movement while bending to your left side. Repeat several times on each side.

Greater challenges

An erect spine, an open chest and awareness of the position of your body and the flow of your energy are the fundamentals of yoga practice. Standing and sitting tall, at all times, will quickly improve your grace and posture and also help to prevent backache and digestive problems, while daily practice of deep breathing with awareness will soon make this your natural way to breathe. These simple practices are also the basis from which you can go on to develop more challenging yoga poses.

24 Adapted easy tree pose

This is a balancing pose requiring good posture, steady deep breathing, stillness and focus. Start with the simpler versions of this pose and work up to the classical pose in your own time. All balancing poses create inner calm and poise as well as physical stillness. Standing tall and balanced becomes more difficult as the baby grows out to the front, so it is important to develop your balancing muscles from the beginning of your pregnancy in order to maintain your grace and poise throughout it.

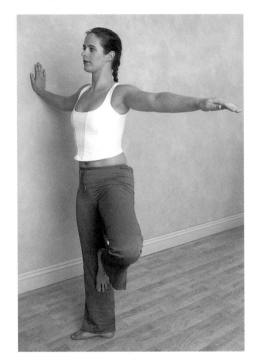

◁ 1 Stand with a wall on your right side. Stretch both arms to the sides at shoulder level. Rest your right hand against the wall for balance. Stand tall with chest open and coccyx tucked under. Bend your left knee and balance on your right foot. Now place your left sole against the inside of your right leg and bring your left knee to the side, opening up the left hip without compromising your erect posture. The aim is to get your knee out to the left so that you can push your sole high up against the right groin, without tilting your pelvis. Practise on one side then the other.

CAUTION
Make sure you keep your base foot straight and resist swaying to the side of your standing leg.

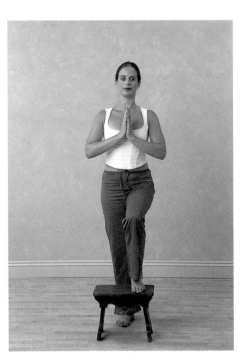

△ **2** Leave the wall and place a low stool in front of you. Place your left foot on the stool and bring your palms together in Namaste, the prayer position, in front of your sternum. Stand tall and gaze at a point in front of you, breathing steadily and deeply.

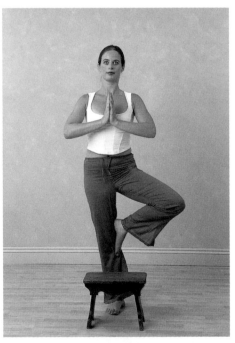

△ **3** Take your left foot off the stool and place the sole against your inner right leg. Use your left hand to help you find a good position for your foot, then return to the Namaste position and your steady gaze with deep breathing. Come out of the position smoothly.

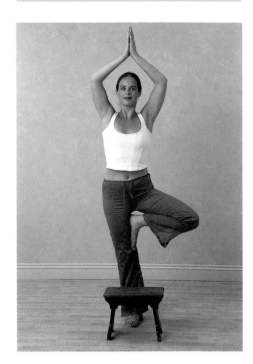

△ **4** This is the classical pose. Place your heel against the groin with the knee out to the side. Focus on your breath and then join your palms together high above your head. Take a few good breaths while in this position, and then relax.

25 Pushing hands

It is fun to practise yoga with a friend, so that you can help each other with your posture. Of course, you can also use a wall if you wish.

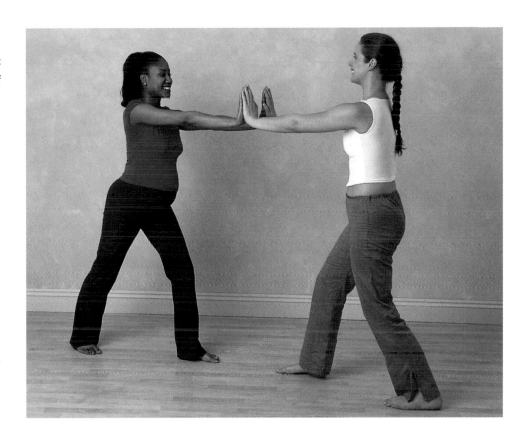

▷ Stand tall, with arms outstretched and palms together. Each person takes a step forward with one leg (you can use either the same or the opposite leg to your partner). Keeping upright, with your hips facing forward, press your palms against those of your partner. Use comfortable pressure as you press, and, as you do so, breathe as deeply as you can and feel the involvement of your abdominal muscles. Change legs and repeat.

26 Classical "cobbler's pose"

This seated position was traditionally used by cobblers and tailors, who needed to use both their hands and also hold things between their feet, and we can still benefit from it today. Many Western women have tight ligaments in the groin and pelvic area, through frequent sitting in a chair or car. It is important to stretch this whole area for ease in giving birth.

Practise sitting on the floor instead of lounging in an easy chair whenever you can – to watch TV, read or chat, for example – and this open position will soon become familiar and comfortable. Place cushions under your knees to begin with, until the groin ligaments stretch and relax naturally. Sit against a wall, or piece of solid furniture, until you can hold your spine erect without discomfort. Once this position feels easy and natural you can also use it to meditate on your baby or to practise deep breathing.

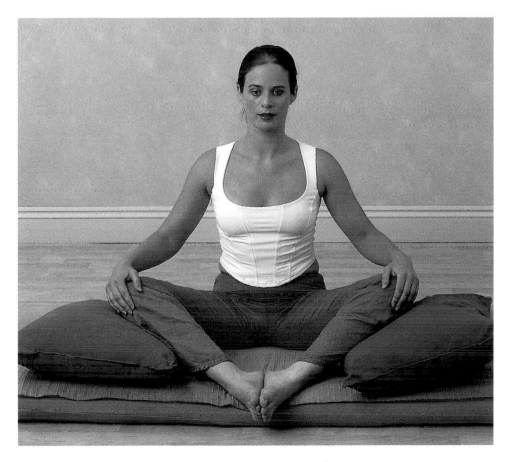

CAUTION
Ligaments need to be stretched gradually and naturally without hurry or forcing. This is especially true during pregnancy, when special hormones gradually soften your ligaments so that they will stretch naturally to allow your baby to be born.

Make yoga a part of your life

There is no special time to practise deep breathing, stretching, relaxation, meditation or quietly observing your body, your feelings and your thoughts. All these are yoga practices that you can do as you go about your daily activities, or fit into those moments when you create a pause between one activity and the next. A few minutes of yogic awareness, frequently repeated, becomes a habit that gradually builds up good health, positive feelings and a clear and focused mind.

27 Sitting position for relaxation and alternate nostril breathing

During the day, you should take a few moments to sit and breathe deeply between one task and the next. Make a conscious decision to change your focus from outer activity to inner silence, so that this becomes a regular rhythm.

Place a comfortable, upright chair, preferably with arms, in a convenient place in your home or office and practise getting into and out of it while keeping your spine stretched and aligned. This may be easy now, but it will become more challenging as your baby grows and the extra weight pulls your lower back into an exaggerated arch, a prime cause of backache. You may need to adjust your sitting position by placing a small cushion between your lumbar arch and the chair, or a stool or cushion under your feet so that they do not hang down without support. If your chair has no arms, place your hands palms up in your lap, or palms down on your thighs.

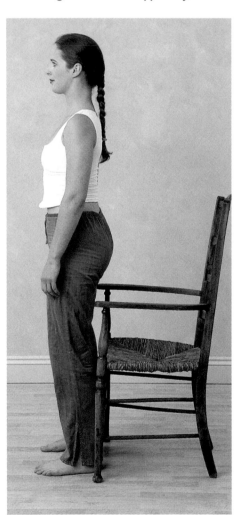

△ **1** Stand tall in front of your yoga chair, looking ahead with your hands by your side. Your back should be well extended and supportive but relaxed rather than rigid.

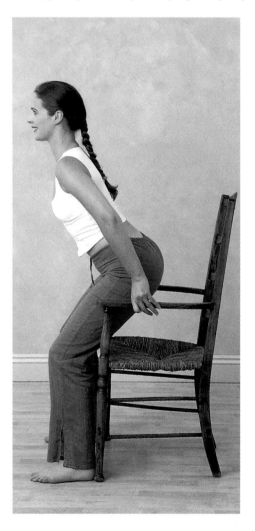

△ **2** Now lower yourself carefully on to the chair, keeping your spine extended and using the arms of the chair for support.

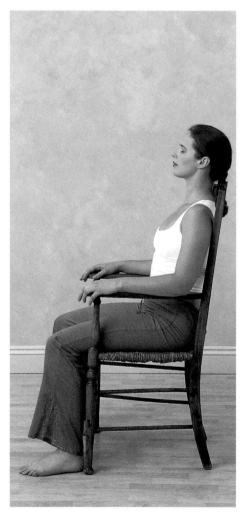

△ **3** Sit upright at the back of the chair, with your spine supported. Place your forearms on the chair arms and plant your feet hip-width apart on the floor. Breathe slowly and deeply with eyes closed, moving your focus inward. While in this seated position, practise Alternate Nostril Breathing (6).

28 Stretch the spine with deep breathing

Your kitchen is an excellent place to practise yogic stretches, as it will probably have a work surface that is a useful height, and maybe a high chair or stool. And you can stretch while waiting for the kettle to boil. The whole body benefits from this sequence. Your legs and feet are strengthened in preparation for carrying the extra weight of your growing baby, and the spine is extended to make more room and to allow for deeper breathing and better digestion. The upper back and neck are freed from any build-up of tension and your grace and balance are enhanced.

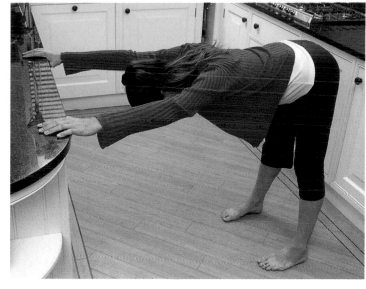

▷ **1** Place your hands on a work surface and walk away from it, bending at the hips until your trunk is stretched out at a right angle to your hips, with as much space as possible between your ribs and your hips. Keep your neck and head level, with your ears between your arms, and your feet a little more than hip-width apart. Breathe slowly and deeply in this position, feeling the movements of the diaphragm.

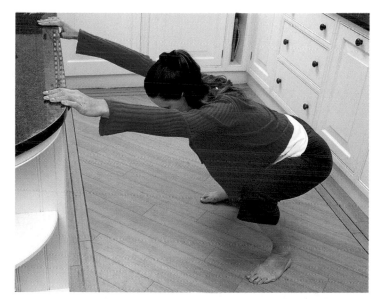

◁ **2** Breathing out, bend your knees into an easy squat without moving your feet. Come back up on an in breath. Repeat.

▷ **3** If you are able to keep your back straight in a full squat, practise closer to the work surface, breathing fully in the pose.

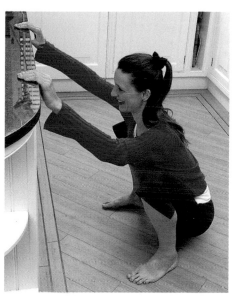

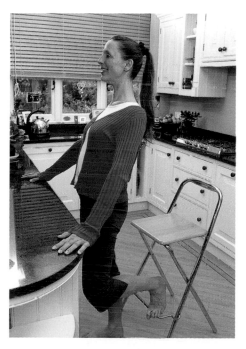

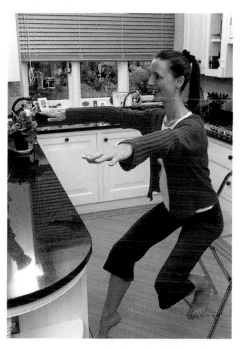

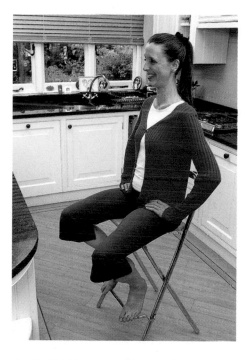

△ **4** Place a high stool or chair behind you to sit on. Stand tall with your hands on the work surface. Breathe in and take one foot back toward the stool.

△ **5** Raise your arms to shoulder level and breathe out as you lower yourself on to the stool, keeping your spine erect and stretched up.

△ **6** Sit tall on the stool with your hands on your upper thighs and elbows bent to the sides to open your chest and shoulders. Breathe deeply, holding this open position. Stand slowly on an in breath.

relax and meditate with your baby

Focusing upon one thing, so that your heart and mind become peaceful and calm, takes you from deep relaxation into the meditative state. This yogic method is especially fulfilling when you are pregnant, as your baby can become the focus of your meditation. In addition, your baby will benefit enormously from your peaceful state and will relax with you.

This focus on your baby from the very beginning of his or her existence creates a close emotional bond between you even before birth – so that you and your baby are communicating and growing ever closer and more comfortable with each other right from conception. This is especially helpful if you have not had a baby before.

29 Walking meditation

It is important to take a break, with a change of activity and focus, when you have been sitting or doing mental work for a while. Stand up and stretch, then align your spine and go for a gentle walking meditation somewhere quiet, either indoors or outdoors. Your footsteps and breathing will gradually synchronize, taking you deep into yourself and into communion with your baby

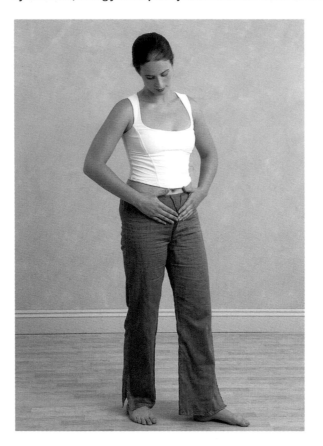

◁ Stand tall and walk very slowly, with short, easy steps. Focus on your baby, placing your hands on your lower abdomen, over your womb. As you breathe in, lift your chest and open your heart space to receive the energy this brings. As you breathe out feel that you are giving this energy, and your love, to your baby. After a few moments, bring your attention slowly back to the outside world. Breathe deeply with a sigh or a yawn, stretch your arms overhead, look all around you and focus on the world outside yourself. Then return to daily life, fully refreshed and at peace.

30 Deep relaxation, watching the flow of the breath

It is easiest to relax completely when lying on your back, either with your feet up the wall or with cushions or a beanbag under your knees. If you plan to relax for more than 10 minutes you may want to cover yourself with a blanket or rug, as your body temperature may drop. Get comfortable and settled, close your eyes and breathe deeply and steadily for a few moments. Allow your mind to rest on the sensations of breathing.

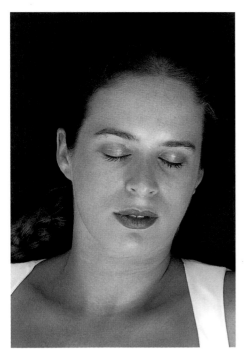

◁ Let your attention follow the passage of air in through your nose, deep into your lungs and out again through your nose in a rhythmic, soothing cycle. When you are ready to get up, breathe strongly and deeply before stretching through your whole body and, finally, opening your eyes.

"I am light with

meditation..."

Douglas Dunn

A sample practice for the early months

1

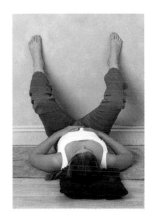

▷ **Feet up the wall sequence (15)**

2

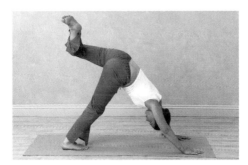

△ **Dog pose (19)**

3

▷ **Grounding (21)**

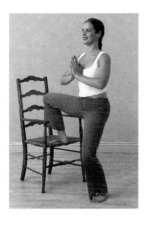

4

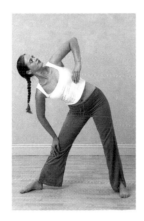

◁ **Triangle sequence (23)**

5

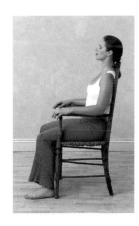

◁ **Sitting position for relaxation and alternate nostril breathing (27)**

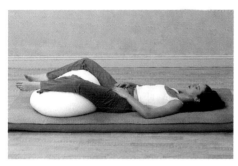

6

△ **Deep relaxation with focused breathing (18)**

Questions and answers

• **I suffer from severe nausea. Is there anything I can do about this?**
Nausea is a common problem while your hormonal system is adjusting to the requirements of pregnancy. It usually eases up after about 12 weeks and may be Nature's way of getting you to slow down until your pregnancy is firmly established. Practise relaxation with slow, gentle breathing, and avoid changing position too quickly. Many women find it helpful to sip milk or nibble dry biscuits, to give something for the stomach to work on between meals.

• **I get a lot of heartburn. What can I do apart from take medicine?**
Avoid rich or spicy foods and large meals. Keep putting bland food, such as a dry biscuit, into your stomach to absorb excess gastric juices. Watch your posture to avoid compression around the waist. Focus on the diaphragm and breathe deeply rather than in the upper chest only. Lean back from the waist with your palms pressed against your lumbar spine.

• **I feel sleepy, lethargic and tired most of the time. Any suggestions?**
This is Nature's way of getting you to rest, and the cure is to do so. Prioritize your activities and cut out the least essential ones to create more space in your life. Establishing a pregnancy takes up a great deal of energy but the good news is that you are likely to feel full of vitality once this early stage has passed.

• **Pregnancy is a totally new experience for me and I am really worried that I may miscarry.**
Breathe deeply and foster feelings of contentment and trust in Nature. Remember that your baby is becoming more firmly established in your body with every week that passes. Trust in the whole process, nurture your mind and body and enjoy regular relaxation practices – stresses of any kind will only increase any chance of miscarriage.

• **I feel anxious because I do not know how to cope with my pregnancy or if I'll be able to cope with my baby when he or she arrives.**
This problem arises because we can feel isolated in modern society. Many of us do not have an extended family on hand to support and advise us through the important stages in our lives, as would have been the case in past generations.

Help and reassurance are available, however. Join an antenatal group and make friends with other mothers-to-be – preferably in your neighbourhood, so you can easily get together to share experiences. Get to know women with babies and children and handle their babies, so that you will feel more confident when your own baby arrives. Joining a special prenatal yoga class or group gives women a regular opportunity to relax and become stronger and more confident. Above all, concentrate on breathing, relaxing – and trusting your inner wisdom.

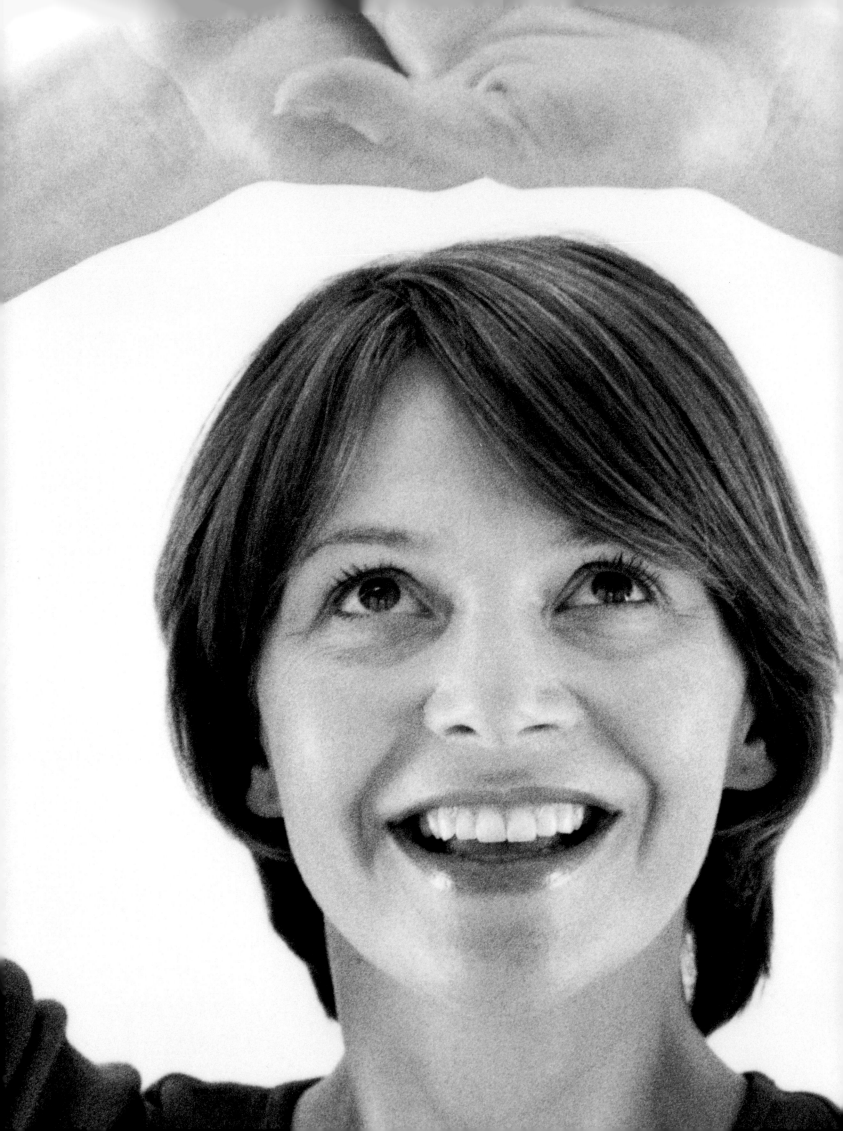

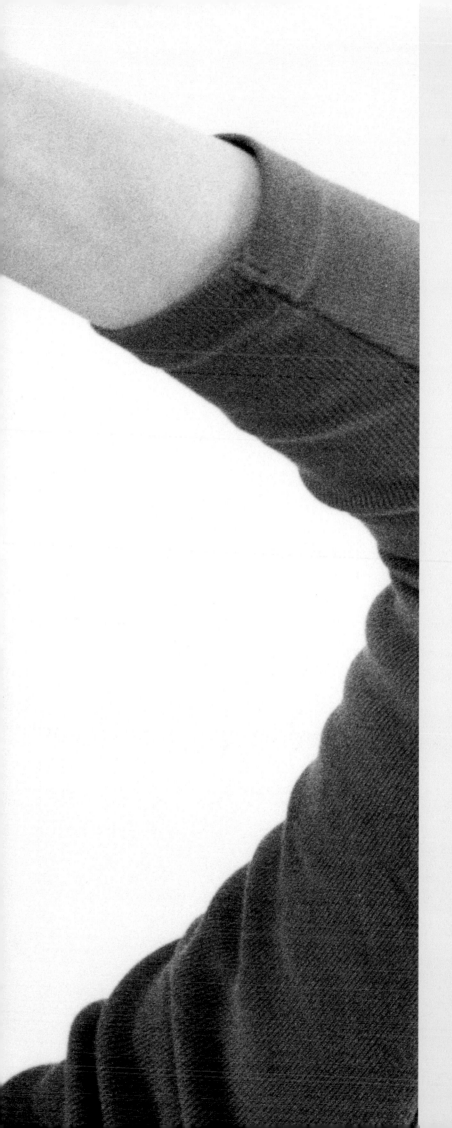

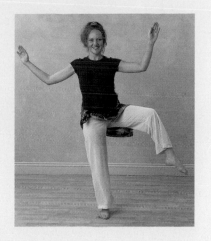

15–30
weeks

Your pregnancy is now firmly established and you should be feeling full of vigour and joy, especially if you have been practising yoga regularly along the lines suggested so far. It is time to focus on building up strength and stamina, on making space to "breathe for two" as your baby grows, and on creating and maintaining the best possible alignment of the spine at all times. Most of all – time to enjoy your pregnancy.

breathing for two

You are likely to be feeling much more energetic during this middle stage, so enjoy your vitality – many of the yoga routines designed for these months are lively, invigorating, almost dance-like. They get your breathing and circulation working optimally and the vigorous arm movements and upward stretches, plus deep breathing, help blood circulate through the abdominal organs and bring fresh, nourishing blood to your baby via the placenta.

31 Sunwheel stretch

This exercise really focuses on upper body stretches to open the chest and loosen the shoulders. The movements wake up the whole of the upper spine and dissolve tightness in the neck, shoulders and arms – this is particularly helpful if you spend a lot of time sitting at a desk or driving a car. These movements also create more space in the abdomen, so that your digestive system has room to function and your baby has room to grow.

You will find at this stage that your balance changes as your abdomen enlarges, so it is important to take your centre of gravity downward, while keeping your spine stretched up and your chest open. This upright, graceful stance will make you feel elegant and confident and also allows more space to be created around the diaphragm, which needs to find room to contract downward so that you are able to breathe really deeply and fully.

▷ **1** Sit with knees a comfortable width apart and feet firmly planted on the floor. Tuck your coccyx under so that your pelvis is level – imagine that the pelvis is a bowl of water and you don't want to spill any of it. Stretch up through your spine from the base to the crown, with your neck long and shoulders relaxed and down. Breathe in deeply to open and lift the chest. Hold the lift as you breathe out, drawing your shoulder blades together with arms relaxed and then pushing the palms down toward the floor with fingers spread wide, to end with straight arms. Repeat, pushing down against imaginary resistance with each breath out and relaxing your hands as you breathe in.

"Oneness of breath and mind... this is called Yoga, integration."

Maitri Upanishad 25

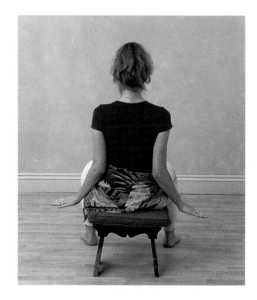

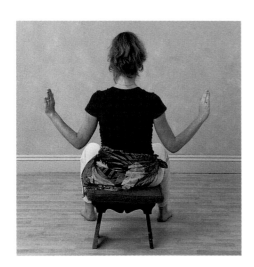

△ **2** Repeat, but this time start with your elbows bent and hands pointing up as you breathe in – this is so that you create a greater push downward as you breathe out. Make your movements graceful and rhythmical, rather like a seated dance.

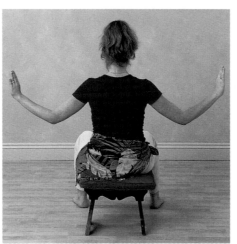

△ **3** Then, on each breath out, push strongly away from you to the sides, with your palms at shoulder level (the picture shows mid-push; you finish the push with straight arms). Engage the muscles around your spine and the back of your waist as you push. Relax as you breathe in. Repeat rhythmically.

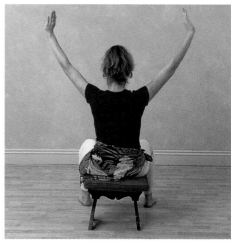

△ **4** On an out breath, stretch your palms to the sides with arms raised as high as you can, engaging your upper arms and back muscles. Finally, repeat the arm movements in reverse order, moving down until your arms are beside you. Repeat the whole sequence several times.

32 Swing high, swing low

This movement should be done rhythmically and with enthusiasm. It loosens up all the joints from your heels to your fingertips and blows away the cobwebs from your mind.

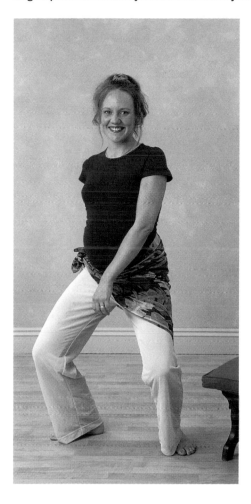

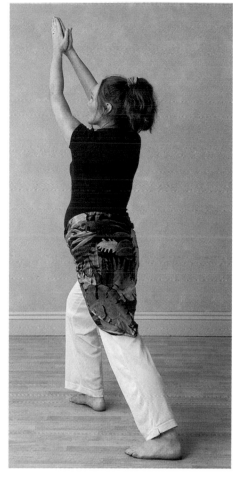

◁ **1** Stand with feet comfortably apart and knees well bent, and rotate your upper body from side to side, making sure your arms are loose and relaxed. Keep your spine upright, your hips and legs steady and your centre of gravity low.

◁ **2** Now stretch your arms right up to the right and clap your hands. Then sink into the previous position before stretching up to the left to clap your hands. Keep breathing deeply and vigorously as you alternately sink and relax then stretch to each side in turn.

33 Centring down

Getting your legs, rather than your lower back, to support your increasing weight and bulk is probably the most important postural adjustment that you can make during your pregnancy because it will save you from backache. Your womb is situated in the lower abdomen, which is held in place by the spine at the back, the pelvic girdle below and the hips on each side, so it has nowhere to expand as your baby grows except upward and forward. Any upward growth is constrained by your digestive organs and diaphragm, so most of the bulk has to move forward. This extra weight should flow downward through strong and well-toned legs, restoring your vital balance and centre of gravity.

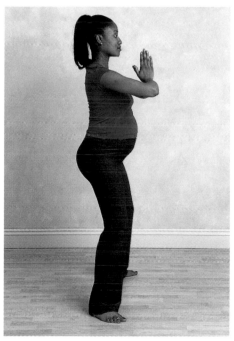

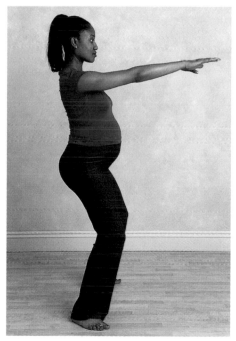

△ **1** Stand with legs a comfortable width apart, feet firmly planted and knees loose. Stretch your spine upwards, taking your weight downwards through your legs. Press your palms together at throat height with elbows out to the sides. Breathe in and expand the lungs at the back by opening your back ribs more.

△ **2** As you breathe out stretch your arms forward and bend deeply at the knees. Hold a moment, then breathe in again. Repeat often.

Yoga and movement

When you are pregnant it is better to move through a variety of yogic positions, in a type of yogic dance, than to hold each position separately. This encourages deeper breathing, which is important as your breath provides oxygen for your baby's metabolism as well as your own. The yogic dance creates more flexibility in all your joints, making you feel loose and limber despite the added weight and bulk of your growing baby. Moving the spine rhythmically in all directions takes pressure off the lower back and strengthens all the muscles that hold the spine in alignment. Moving with knees well bent ensures that you avoid arching your back and that your spine and pelvis remain perfectly aligned. Your shoulders and neck should remain relaxed throughout.

34 Pat on the back

This free and rhythmic swinging movement loosens the tensions that so readily gather around the upper spine and shoulders after sitting. It also eases stresses in the joints of the hands and arms.

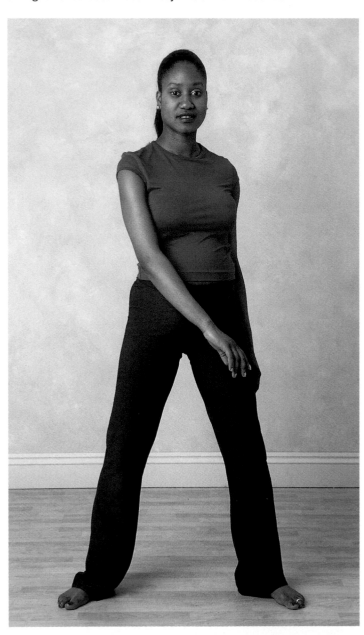

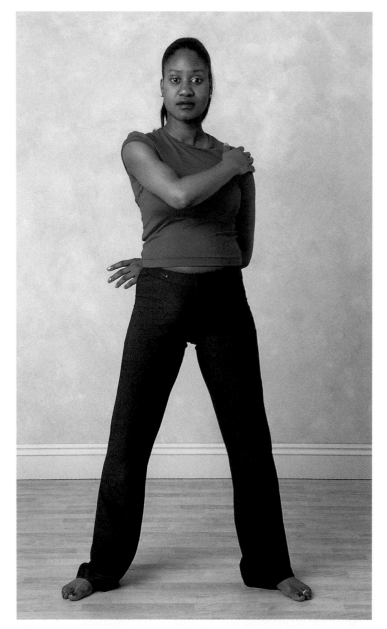

△ **1** Stand tall, with knees very loose and coccyx tucked under. Swing your upper body from the shoulders, letting your arms and hands hang freely. Swing from one side to the other, but face to the front – your head and hips do not move.

△ **2** Repeat this relaxed swinging movement, but this time bend your elbows so that you bring one hand right up and slightly over your shoulder, as though almost patting yourself on the back, and the other arm around to the back of your waist.

35 Ball of energy (1)

Imagine that you are playing with a huge, soft, invisible ball of energy. You create it by rubbing your palms briskly together, rather like rubbing two sticks together to create a flame. Then separate your hands a little before bringing them closer together in a pumping or kneading movement to enlarge your energy ball. Use your imagination and sense of touch, feeling that you are actually plumping up the ball of energy, tossing it from one hand to the other and holding it lightly between your fingertips as it grows and grows.

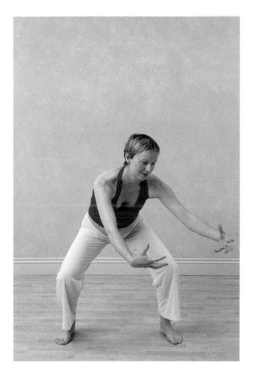

△ **1** Keeping your knees well bent and spine stretched, bend forward with your ball of energy, holding it lightly between your open palms.

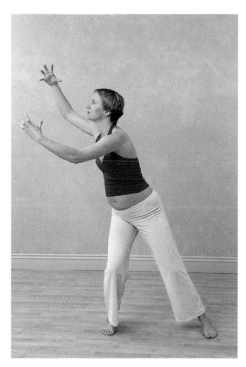

△ **2** Now toss the invisible ball of energy to the side, twisting your body in a wide movement, but without moving your feet at all.

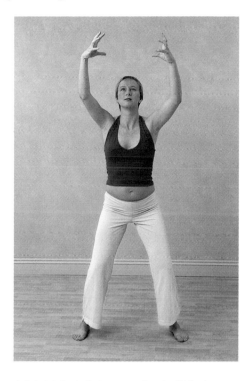

△ **3** Catch the ball above your head, with both arms. Keep your arms and your legs slightly bent, and feel that you are centred around the naval area.

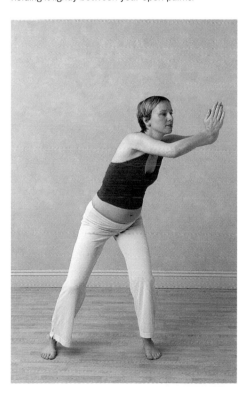

△ **4** Compress your ball, then roll it across your body, first on one side then on the other, twisting your body in a wide movement, from a strong base.

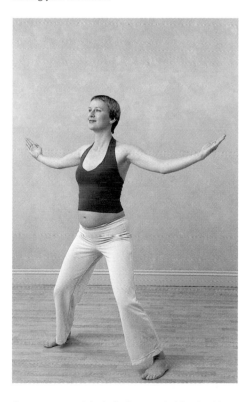

△ **5** Now expand the ball of energy, holding it with your arms wide to the sides and opening your chest. Your base should be strong, with knees slightly bent.

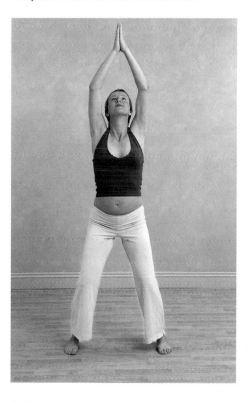

△ **6** Be inventive and lively as you continue to play with the ball, stretching and moving in all directions. When you have done enough, hold it between your palms and gently squeeze it until it gets smaller and smaller and disappears between your joined palms.

Gentle twists and shoulder stretches

Vigorous exercise with arm movements and deep, natural breathing is a good way of keeping healthy, strong and supple while you are carrying your baby. It gets your circulation going, makes you feel great and relieves any strain, tension and tiredness that may have been building up in your neck and shoulders. It also exercises the muscles of the trunk and spine. These kinds of invigorating movements require both concentration and focus. They are most effective if you keep your knees bent throughout.

36 Thunder claps

These positions work the muscles across the chest and upper spine to lift the sternum and open the chest for deeper breathing, as well as opening and rotating the shoulder joints and strengthening the arms to relieve stiffness and tension. The pectoral muscles across the upper chest can become shortened if we slouch forward, especially when sitting at a desk or table and leaning upon our elbows. Let the vigorous rhythm of this exercise do the stretching for you, even if you can't clap behind your back at first. You will soon loosen up with frequent practice and enjoy the feeling of openness in the chest.

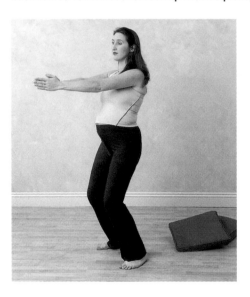

◁ **1** Stand tall through your spine, but with knees well bent and feet more than hip-width apart. Stretch your arms out to the front and clap your hands at shoulder level, reaching forward to open the back of the shoulders without moving the spine.

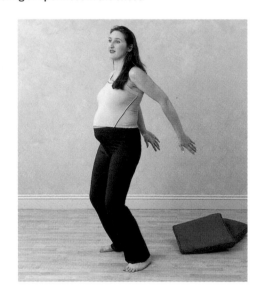

◁ **2** Now take your hands behind you and as high up as you can, to open the shoulder joints at the front and stretch the pectoral muscles across the upper chest. Bring your palms together to clap, straightening your arms if you can.

37 Disco twist

This is a rhythmic, twisting movement done with feet wide and knees well bent. Get into the swing of it, following your natural rhythm, and really get your breath and bloodstream moving. Stop as soon as you feel out of breath and rest in the starting position before moving on to the next exercise.

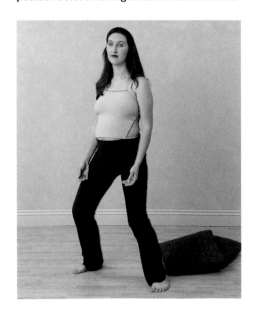

◁ **1** Stand with knees springy and loose and feet comfortably apart, arms relaxed.

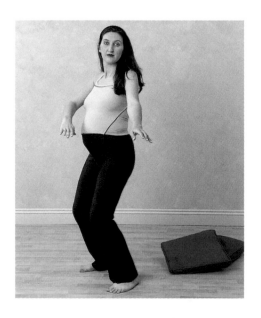

◁ **2** Lift your chest and twist your upper body to the left, and also swing your arms and hands to the left. Bend your knees a little more to dip to the left, lift up again and twist to the right and repeat. Keep your coccyx tucked under, your spine upright and your legs springy as you twist from one side to the other.

38 Crossovers

These wide, sweeping movements combine stretching with a bending and twisting of the trunk. They require mental focus and deep, rhythmical breathing, and will fill you with energy, so practise them regularly. Circle your arms boldly, as though they have flags attached and you want to be seen from a distance. Crossovers require good co-ordination and are best done naturally and vigorously, without too much thought.

Start out by doing the sequence as a plain twist-and-stretch, feeling the lengthening in each side of your body as you alternate arms. Then build up to a much more fluid, wider circling movement, by stretching up higher, bending lower at the knees and twisting more deeply. Eventually, you should feel that as soon as you reach the maximum stretch on one arm, the other arm is sinking down to create another circle overlapping the previous one.

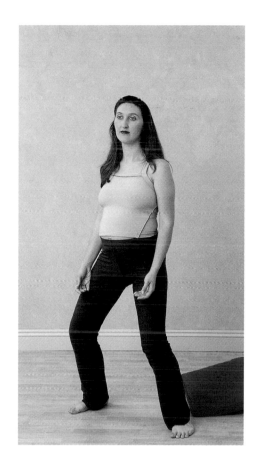

△ **1** Stand with knees springy and loose and feet a comfortable width apart – as you did in Step 1 of the Disco Twist (37).

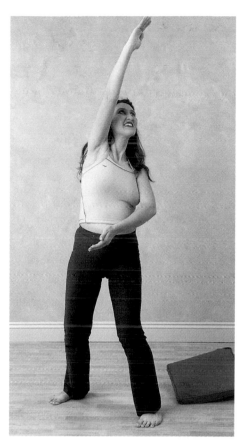

△ **2** Slowly twist the upper body to the left as you raise your right arm in front of you and stretch it up high. Look up at it.

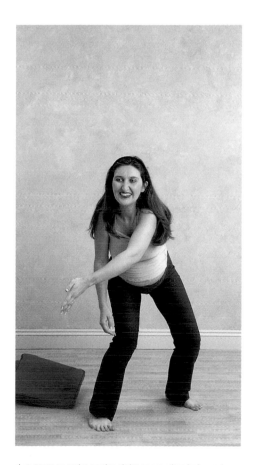

△ **3** Start to twist to the right as you begin lowering your right arm in a circle behind you. Keep the chest open and your knees well bent. At the same time start to take your left arm in front of you.

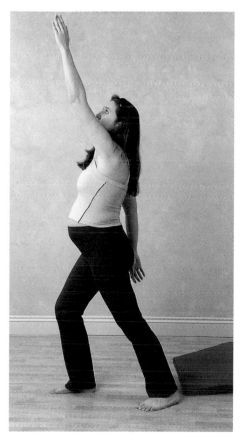

△ **4** When your left arm is stretched right up, look at your left hand. Try to make as straight a line as possible from your back heel to the very tip of the middle finger of your stretched hand.

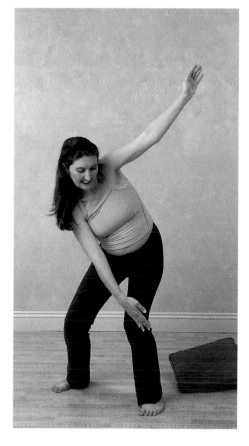

△ **5** Lower your left arm behind you as you start to twist to the left, and bring your right arm through to the front and across your body, ready to raise it again to complete the double circle. Repeat several times.

The three movements of the pelvis

Flexibility in the pelvis is natural in young children, and also in adults who live in traditional societies without the comforts and technology that we take for granted. But our sophisticated, Western way of life inhibits this flexibility, from schooldays onwards. We don't squat down to wash clothes or prepare food. Instead, we spend most of our waking hours in one form of chair or another while we chat, read, use the computer, and even while travelling. In order to regain our innate grace and suppleness, and to maintain it throughout our lives, we need to relearn the natural ways of holding and moving our bodies. Flexibility in the spine, hips and pelvis is especially important during pregnancy, as it alleviates many common discomforts, such as backache, sciatica and cramps, and also prepares the body for active, easy birthing.

> "How long will you keep expecting answers from outside? Just go inside."
>
> *Frederick Leboyer*

39 Seated pelvic rolls

Your lower abdominal muscles and the long transverse abdominal muscles (at the sides of the trunk) need to be strong and active, or they fail to play their part in supporting the weight of the body and leave your lower back muscles to carry the whole load. This exercise is a good way of strengthening both these sets of muscles.

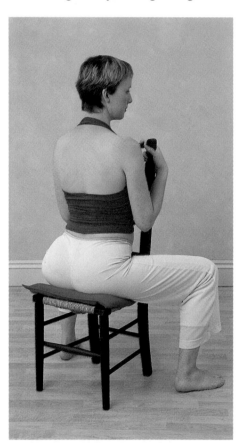

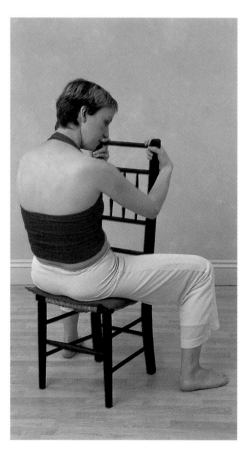

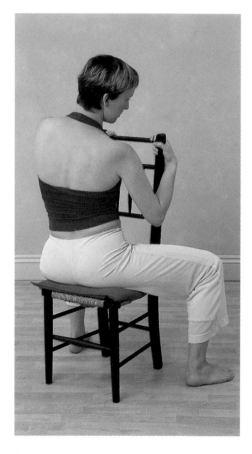

△ **1** Sit squarely in a sturdy, upright chair, facing the back of the chair. Place your sitting bones near the front of the seat and hold on to the back of the chair for support. Arch your lower back strongly, lowering the front rim of your pelvis forward and bringing your abdomen closer to the chair. Feel the muscles of your spine contracting strongly as the abdominal muscles relax.

△ **2** Reverse this movement by tilting your pelvis back to lift the front rim of the pelvis. Stretch and relax your lower spine. The lower abdominal muscles are now contracting strongly.

△ **3** Now contract the long muscles on your right side, while consciously relaxing and stretching the ones on the left. This will lift your right hip up toward your right ribs, so that you are sitting on one side of the lower pelvis (your left sitting bone). Repeat this on the other side. Gradually combine these movements into a flowing, clockwise roll. Then repeat in an anti-clockwise direction.

40 Standing pelvic roll

This is a stronger, standing version of Seated Pelvic Rolls (39). It can be practised easily in any spare moment. If the abdomen feels distended and crowded by the growing baby, a few pelvic rolls can quickly create more space and relieve uncomfortable pressure. Placing your hands on your hips helps you to focus on the pelvic girdle and become more aware of its range of movement.

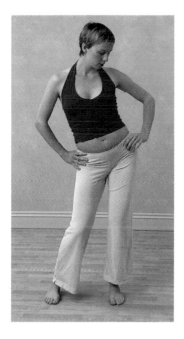

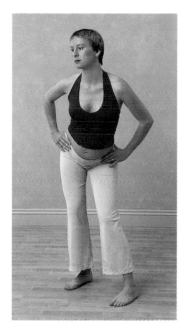

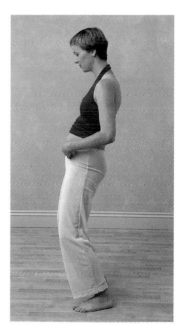

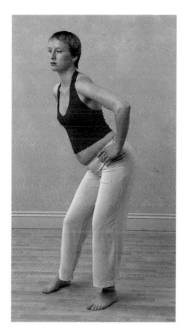

△ **1** Stand with feet apart and knees well bent and springy. Place your hands on the front of your hip bones. Keep your whole spine stretched up from the base and through your neck and shoulders to the crown. Tilt your pelvis up on the left side so that you contract the transverse abdominal muscles on the left side and relax them on the right side. Don't move above the waist.

△ **2** Now drop your pelvis on the left side and tilt it up on the right side. Practise these two movements until they are smooth and flowing.

△ **3** Stand up straight again and roll the rim of the pelvis forward and upward, tucking your coccyx under and lengthening and relaxing through your lower spine. Avoid clenching your buttocks, as you allow the lower abdominal muscles to stretch with the forward movement.

△ **4** Tilt the rim of your pelvis down and back to arch your lower back. These four movements make up the pelvic roll. Continue round clockwise – left hip up, pelvic rim up, right hip up, pelvic rim down – in a smooth, rolling movement. Finish with the same number of anti-clockwise rolls.

41 Jump for joy

This is an exuberant movement, celebrating the lightness and grace in your legs and hips. Feel yourself bursting with energy and full of the joys of life as you open your hips and chest wide, affirming your trust in a world that welcomes the baby that you are now carrying within you. You can even include a light jump in the air if you feel like it.

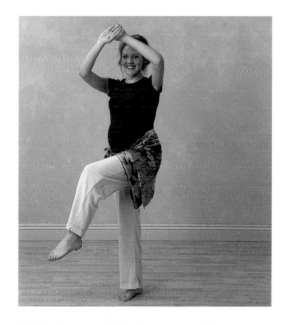

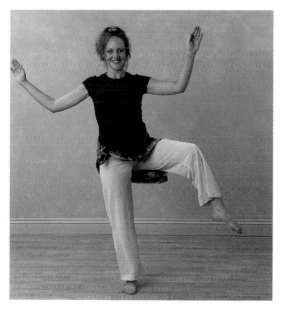

△ **1** Stand on your right leg, keeping your right knee relaxed. As you raise your left knee in front of you to hip height, bring your elbows high and wide, with the backs of your hands above your face.

△ **2** Open your left hip to swing your left knee to the side at hip height, flinging your arms wide, still at shoulder height. Step down on to your left side and bring your right knee up to repeat on the other side. Keep your arms circling round.

Gaining strength and stamina

The following movements have isometric qualities: that is, one set of muscles contracts strongly to push against a second set that are resisting the push. The result, with practice, is that both sets of muscles get stronger by pushing against each other. There is also a centring and stabilizing effect, as the two-way push ripples throughout the whole body. Each strong pushing movement should be balanced by a letting-go pose, so that muscular strength is built up rather than muscular tension. Isometric exercise helps posture, breathing and spinal alignment. It builds strength symmetrically, which is especially important during pregnancy.

42 Swing and release

In this vigorous exercise, the palms are pressed firmly together to strengthen the muscles of the hands and arms, and especially the muscles that lie each side of the upper spine. Strength here makes it easy to maintain a good upright posture through the spine and neck, so that the circulation of the blood and the messages passing along the nervous system can flow freely through the neck and trunk. Raising the arms while pressing the hands together strengthens the muscles at the sides of the body and lifts the sternum for deeper breathing.

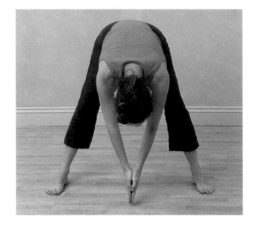

◁ **1** Stand with your feet a comfortable width apart and your knees bent but relaxed and loose. Bring your palms together and bend forward from the hips so that your fingertips touch the floor. Breathe out in this position.

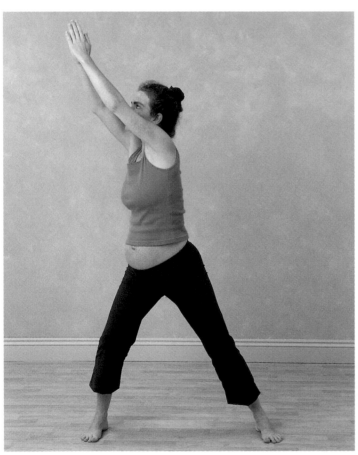

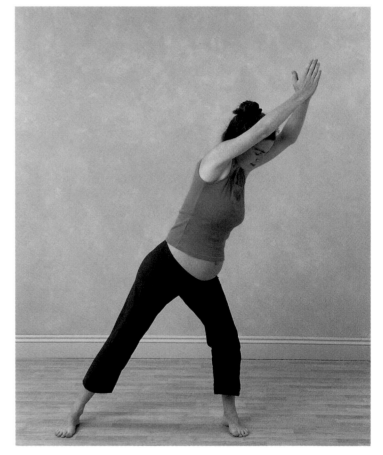

△ **2** Stretch your arms forward, pushing the palms hard against each other and engaging the muscles of your upper back for lifting. Breathe in strongly, raising your head, arms and trunk up and to the right side, twisting the spine to the right from the waist upward. Hold this position for a few seconds, pressing your palms together and feeling your muscles engaging all along your arms and upper spine.

△ **3** On a strong breath out through the mouth in a "HAH" sound, drop back to your starting position with your knees well bent. Keep your hands together and strong, like a knife slicing through bread. Let go of all effort as you breathe in and out to relax in the starting position, before breathing in again strongly to repeat the upward stretch and pushing movements to the left side. Repeat a few times.

43 Push and release

Here, two different isometric pushing movements are counter-balanced by the same open and surrendering pose. This is an important principle in everyday life as well as in yoga practice. We should always relax between activities in order to dissolve any physical, emotional or mental tensions before they can take a hold. In this way we build up our strength and stamina rather than depleting our reserves.

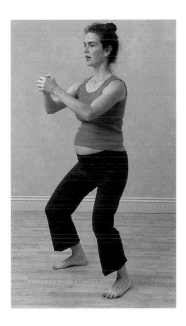

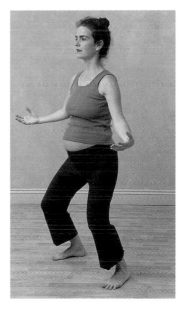

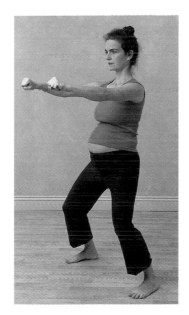

△ **1** Stand with your spine erect, coccyx tucked under, pelvis level and knees well bent. Clasp your hands at chest level and push one hand hard against the other for two strong breaths in and out.

△ **2** Breathe in, then, with a voiced-out breath "aaah", open your arms to the side in a surrendering gesture. Keep the chest open and the back straight. Rest in this position and take a deep breath, relaxing the facial muscles.

△ **3** Bring your arms straight out in front of you and make fists. Push your fists forward, opening and stretching in your back and maintaining balance by using your lower abdominal and front thigh muscles. Then relax as before in the surrender position. Repeat these movements several times.

44 Hip openers in pairs

Two people exercising together can be good fun, but you will also help each other to develop strength and stamina and to improve muscle tone. Be careful to judge your partner's strength and balance – it is easier to work with a partner who is roughly the same height and weight as you are. Some of these positions can also be practised on your own, by using a wall to lean against or a strong counter to pull on.

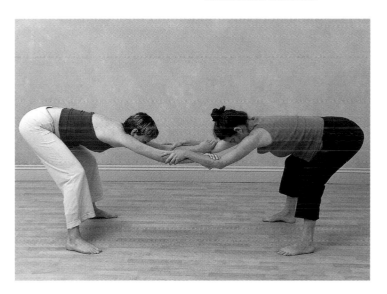

▷ **1** Stand facing each other with feet planted firmly, quite wide apart, and knees loosely bent. Take hold of each other's forearms with a firm grip. Both partners then bend forward at the waist. Adjust your position so that each partner makes a right angle with their legs and trunk. Once settled, start to pull away from each other. Stretch the base of your spine and make space in the lumbar region, wriggling your hips from side to side.

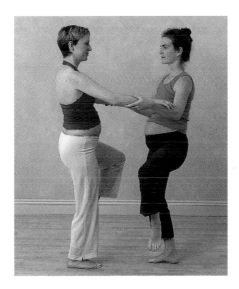

◁ **2** Face to face and gripping each other's forearms, both partners lift their left knees out to the side, opening up the hip joints. This mutual support helps you to keep your balance and also allows you to extend the raised knee further out and back than you could on your own.

▷ **3** After extending the raised knees as far back as possible, both partners land their left foot softly on the floor behind them. Raise the left leg again for another round and repeat a few times. Now change legs to repeat on the other side.

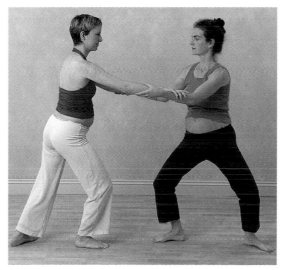

kneeling stretches

Some kneeling positions enable you to build up strength and stamina (to help you carry your baby without getting tired), and kneeling stretches can prevent and ease low back pain. At the same time, kneeling exercises focus upon the birthing muscles. The latter is especially important if this is your first baby, as these muscles will not have been used before. Getting used to a kneeling position for your stretches is an important part of preparing for labour, since many women prefer this position in childbirth.

45 Cat pose

The Cat Pose is traditionally used to loosen all the joints before going into classical yogic seated poses. A simpler version, called the "kitten roll" here, is included as a warm-up. Avoid sagging at the waist by holding your middle spine firmly in line, like a table top, as you move through the rolls.

▷ **1** Kneel on your yoga mat with knees about hip-width apart, so that there is plenty of room for your baby. Place cushions under your knees, if you like. Sit back on your heels and, without lifting your buttocks, stretch your arms out in front, about shoulder-width apart. Crawl forward with your fingers while anchoring your buttocks on to your heels. Feel the stretch through your spine and breathe slowly into this stretch to loosen any tension in your back, hips or shoulders.

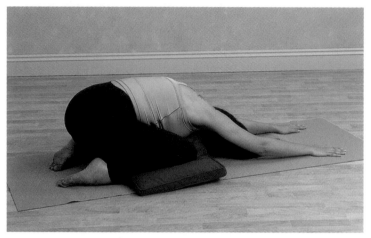

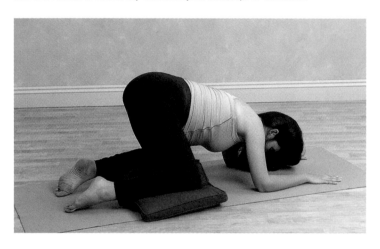

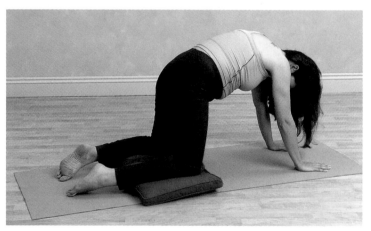

△ **2** For the "kitten roll", sit back on your heels before breathing in to bring your weight forward on to your elbows. Lift your shoulders as you breathe out to arch your spine and tuck your coccyx under before rolling back on to your heels. Repeat the roll several times, and as you do so, focus your attention on feeling the stretch at the back of your waist.

△ **3** For the "cat roll", bring your weight forward on to spread palms as you breathe in, so that your shoulders are directly above your wrists, your arms are straight but not locked at the elbow and your back is flat like a table top. This is the classic Cat Pose. Breathe out to arch and stretch your spine before sitting back on your heels, again, trying not to move your hands. Breathe in to repeat the rolling movement.

46 Hip and knee circles

These circles are practised while in the Cat Pose (45). They loosen tightness in the hip joints, can relieve cramps in the groin and increase the circulation of blood around the abdomen and pelvis.

▷ Place yourself in the Cat Pose (45), with your weight evenly distributed and your back and head held firmly in line. Raise your right knee from the floor, keeping it bent at a right angle, and move it around in small circles parallel to the floor so that you are rotating the hip joint. After circling clockwise and anti-clockwise, repeat this sequence of movements on the left side.

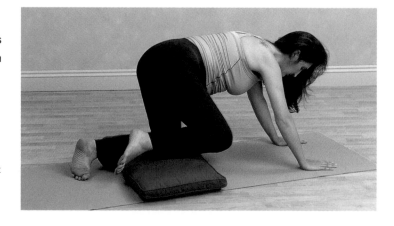

47 Shoulder and elbow circles

These circles are great for relieving tension in the neck and shoulders, stretching the pectoral muscles and opening the chest for deeper breathing. Both exercise 46 and this exercise provide the same benefits as swimming movements.

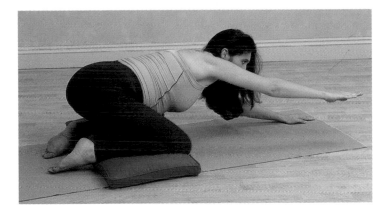

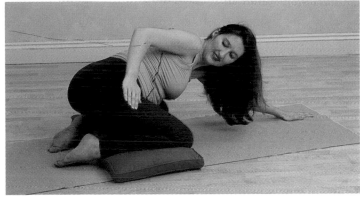

△ **1** Place yourself in the Cat Pose (45) and then sit back on your heels. Keeping your weight evenly balanced, and your spine and head firmly in line, stretch your right arm out in front of you.

△ **2** Bend your right elbow and bring your arm up and back in a circle, turning your head and opening the right side of your chest and your right shoulder. Lift the elbow as high as you can before stretching the arm to the front again. Repeat on the left.

48 Tiger stretch and relax (1)

This is one of the best ways to relieve lower backache and sciatica. This can sometimes become a problem as your pregnancy advances and the weight of your baby presses on the sciatic nerve as it emerges from the lower spine and carries on down your leg. You will need to balance firmly on strong wrists and hands as you raise your leg parallel to the floor.

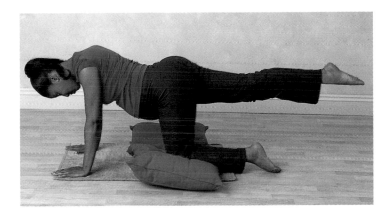

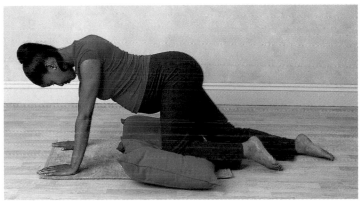

△ **1** Place yourself in the Cat Pose (45) with spine stretched and firm, especially at the waist. Slowly raise your right leg behind you until it is parallel to the floor, neither higher nor lower. Stretch right through your leg and into your toes, and kick away any tension or pressure.

△ **2** Let your leg sink limply to the floor and relax it completely. Maintain your balance and the strength in your spine, but drop your right hip. Shake your leg loosely from hip to toes to release cramps or pressure on the sciatic nerve. Then readjust your position and do the same movements with the left leg.

49 Manual back stretch

As your baby grows it becomes ever more important to relax frequently and to ease away tiredness and tension. A partner or friend can work wonders, simply by gently helping your spine to stretch as you lie comfortably draped over a beanbag or pillows, either on your bed or on the floor. Your helper does not need to be an expert, just intuitive and happy to be guided by you to discover the position where you can relax and breathe most deeply.

▷ Your helper needs to be in a firm, comfortable position, where they do not strain their own back. He or she extends their hands so their fingers trace light pressure either side of your spine as you breathe out. They release pressure on each in breath. Your partner should avoid direct pressure on the spine and check what feels best for you. The aim is to reduce compression and create space and comfort through a gradual deepening of the breath.

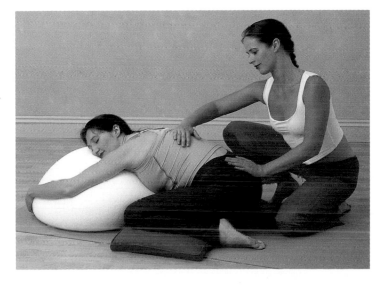

Your birthing muscles

A sphincter is a ring-shaped muscle that acts like a valve by squeezing tightly around the bottom of a tube to keep the contents in. If you want to release the contents, you simply relax the sphincter muscle, or you can get it to push the contents out by controlling the flow with rhythmic pulses. Women have three "tubes" that are either sphincters or are sphincter-like. These open at the base of the body – an area often called the pelvic floor – through the perineum (a mass of muscle that stretches right across the base of the body and holds the abdomen's contents in place.) Each of these openings is controlled by strong muscles, which are:

• the anal tube at the end of our digestive system, which opens to release waste matter. It is found near the base of the spine, at the back of the pelvic floor;

• the urethra – the tube leading from the bladder. This is found close to the pubic bone, at the front of the pelvic floor;

• the muscles each side of the vagina, which can contract and release around the cervix. The cervix thins out during labour to become the birth canal and let your baby descend through the vagina. Squeezing the vaginal muscles – "pulling up inside" – helps you locate and feel your cervix.

With regular practice, you can learn to contract or relax these muscles at will. This will help you throughout pregnancy (when your baby is pressing down against the pelvic floor), during the birth (to help control the baby's movement down through the birth canal), and after the birth (to restore perineal muscle tone as quickly as possible, thus avoiding many common postnatal problems).

exercising the birthing muscles

Yogic philosophy maintains that energy follows thought. So focusing on muscle groups that we usually ignore helps to bring movement to the area and encourages awareness, which leads in turn to control of those muscles. Using the breath intensifies

THE BIRTHING MUSCLES

The pelvic area at around mid-term
Note how the baby presses against the internal organs shown

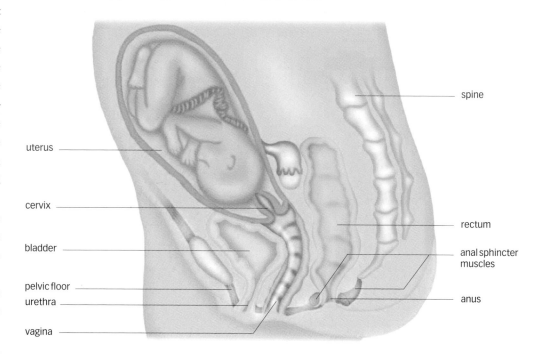

- spine
- uterus
- cervix
- rectum
- bladder
- anal sphincter muscles
- pelvic floor
- urethra
- anus
- vagina

The perineum
(seen from below)

The red, striated areas are muscle

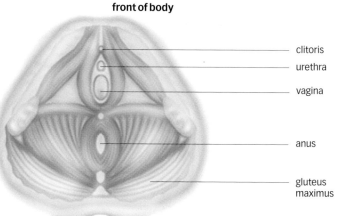

front of body

- clitoris
- urethra
- vagina
- anus
- gluteus maximus

back of body

the muscular action. Yogic actions are never mechanical because you are using your breath and awareness simultaneously with the contraction and relaxation of the muscles. By connecting breath with muscular action you are toning, in a unique way, the muscles of the perineum, including those that attach it to the pelvis at the front and the lower spine at the back.

Begin your birthing muscle workout with the anal sphincter, contracting and

releasing it in turn. Focus on how this feels, so that you learn to draw in the anus on a breath in and slowly release it on a breath out. Now focus on the sphincter of the urethra, squeezing it in and relaxing it in small, rapid movements. Finally, focus on the vaginal muscles, squeezing them tightly to draw your pelvic floor up and in. You will find that the lower abdomen is also drawn up and inward. These are the "birthing muscles" that you want to strengthen.

50 Pelvic floor stretches

In this modification of the Cat Pose (45) your weight is distributed through your knees and elbows, leaving your lower back and pelvis weightless, released from the constraints of gravity that usually restrict flexibility in this area.

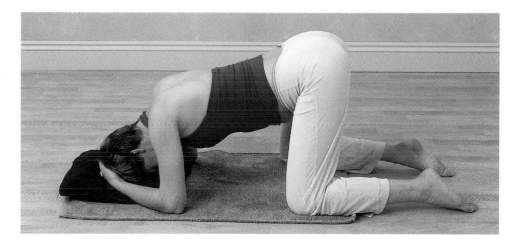

◁ **1** Kneel in the Cat Pose (45), with your knees spread wide enough to accommodate your baby as you lean forward on to your elbows. Place your head on a cushion if it is more comfortable. Distribute your weight evenly between your elbows and your knees, so that your head and neck are comfortable and your coccyx is raised as high as possible. Focus upon your pelvic floor, then exercise the three main birthing "sphincters" one by one, as explained on the opposite page.

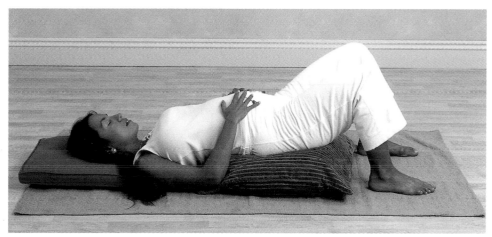

◁ **2** Alternate the kneeling position with this pelvic lift, which uses different sets of inner muscles. Lie on your back with your buttocks on a cushion to raise the pelvis. Keep your knees bent, with feet apart and firmly planted on the floor. Place your hands over your baby to feel the movement as you squeeze the whole pelvic floor in and up. Hold the squeeze for a few breaths to strengthen these muscles, then let go and relax completely. Repeat several times.

51 Supported pelvic floor lift

Your baby needs space to pass down through the vagina. This space is created naturally, as hormones are released during pregnancy to loosen the ligaments that hold your bones in place. This allows your pelvic opening to widen naturally. You can help by relaxing your hip and leg muscles in a wide-legged seated position, reclining comfortably against a beanbag or other support. Do not force yourself, just breathe gently in this position. Once the muscles around the groin have gently relaxed, the ligaments can stretch. In addition, the more relaxed you are the easier it is to practise strengthening the inner muscles of the perineum and vagina.

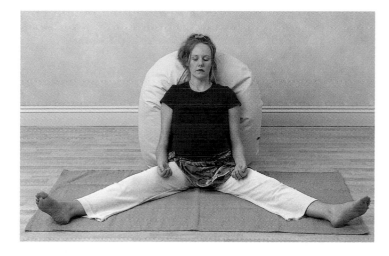

△ **1** Sit with your legs as wide apart as is comfortable for you. Make sure that your spine is well supported, especially at the base. Flex your ankles and stretch through your legs. Lean back and relax in this position. The muscles around the groin area should be especially relaxed, to allow the ligaments to stretch.

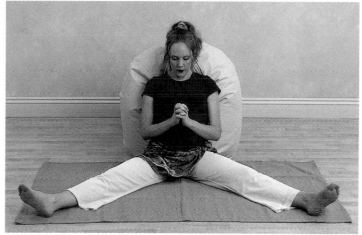

△ **2** Now clasp your hands in front of you at chest height, breathing in as you press your palms firmly together, and at the same time contract the muscles of the perineum and vagina. Hold this contraction for a breath or two, and then relax completely before repeating.

seated stretches

These easy stretches can be done at any time, sitting on a chair or on the floor with your back upright and legs uncrossed. The more you practise, the more flexible and relaxed your whole body will become. If you have to spend hours in front of a computer or driving, for example, try to stretch regularly. You should, of course, be working your inner muscles in the lower abdominal and pelvic area while seated throughout the day. One of the skills that comes with regular yoga practice is the ability to work one area of the body quite strongly while keeping all the other parts completely relaxed.

52 Neck rolls

Tension is apt to build up around the neck and shoulders when you sit and concentrate for any length of time, whether travelling or working at a desk. You can prevent this build-up by being aware of your posture, and by stopping for a short break whenever you can.

▷ Sit erect on an upright chair, maintaining the stretch through your spine as you relax your arms and shoulders. Sit with knees wide and feet planted firmly on the floor, resting your hands comfortably on your thighs. Relax your neck muscles and bring your chin forward, lengthening the back of your neck, then round to your right shoulder. Bring your chin forward again then round to your left shoulder. Repeat gently, with relaxed breathing.

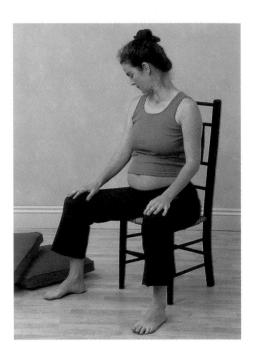

53 Chest expander

This energizing exercise strengthens the muscles that hold your upper spine in place, so it is excellent for improving your posture, as well as increasing your lung capacity for deeper breathing. Try it when you are feeling mentally tired.

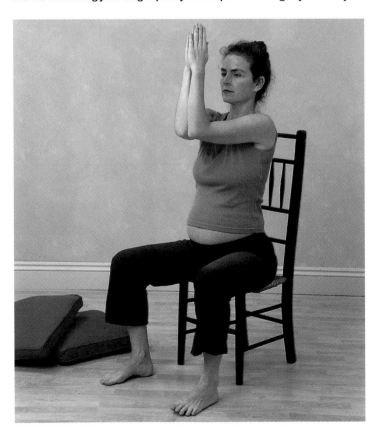

△ **1** Sit upright, with knees wide and feet firmly planted on the floor. Raise your elbows to shoulder height. As you breathe out press your forearms and palms together in front of your face.

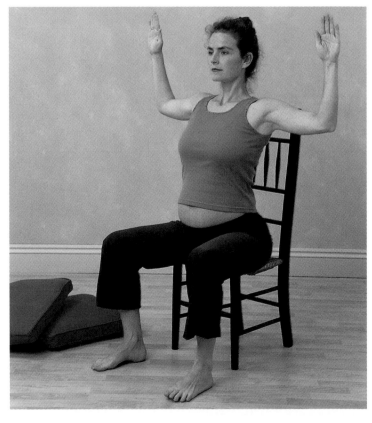

△ **2** As you breathe in take your elbows high and back, squeezing your shoulder blades together, lifting your sternum and stretching your pectoral muscles across your upper chest. Bring your elbows forward again. Repeat several times.

54 Seated side stretch

This exercise prevents and alleviates heartburn. It opens the sides of the body to make more room in the abdomen for better functioning of the diaphragm and the digestive organs. It also gives your developing baby more room to move around.

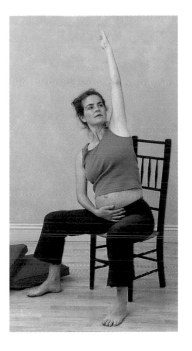

◁ **1** Sit on a firm chair with knees wide and feet on the floor. Bring your left arm out to the side and up overhead, stretching your whole left side. Resting your right elbow on your right thigh, turn your head to look up at your outstretched hand and breathe deeply into the stretched side, holding the position. Repeat on the other side.

▷ **2** For a stronger stretch, place your right ankle on your left thigh then raise your right arm. Hold your foot with your left hand, your ankle flexed and in line as you drop your right knee to the side. Stretch your right arm up. Hold, breathing deeply into the stretched side. Repeat on the other side.

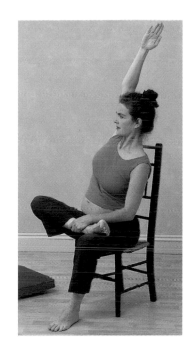

55 Seated stretches in pairs

This lively sequence is fun to do and really gets your energy flowing and blood circulation moving. If you are different heights, then the shorter partner can sit on a cushion to even things out.

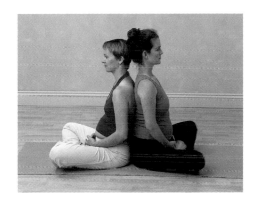

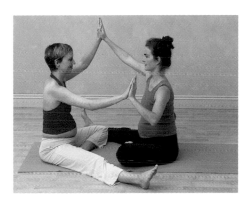

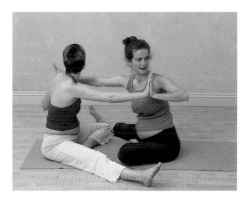

△ **1** Sit back to back with legs crossed and spines pulled upward. Lean on each other just enough to increase awareness of the position of your spines, so that you can both adjust your alignment. Breathe deeply and notice how you start to breathe together.

△ **2** Face each other with right legs straight and left knees bent (left feet against right thighs). Sit up tall with your palms pressed against your partner's palms. Circle your hands out to the sides and in again. Change legs and repeat.

△ **3** Keep in the same position, but this time both partners use isometric pressure on each other's palms to rotate the trunk, twisting first to one side and then the other. Look over your shoulder to take the twist through your upper spine and neck.

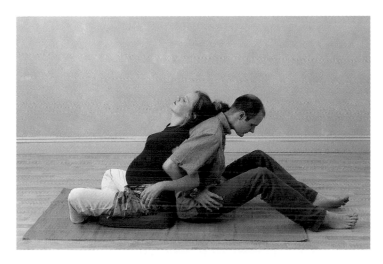

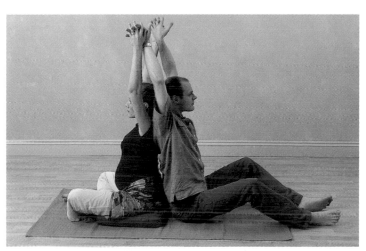

△ **4** Sit back to back with your legs crossed or knees comfortably bent. Link arms and rock back and forth, so that one partner folds forward as the other stretches backward. Keep your spines in contact while rocking.

△ **5** Hold each other's hands, then stretch your arms out to the sides and up overhead to maintain a stretch in the sides of your trunk. Go gently and learn to sense what the other person needs – no force, pulling or pushing.

lying down stretches

When you are tired – or after your standing, kneeling and sitting exercises – you can lie down to relax and also stretch, so that you are still gaining strength and flexibility while the floor supports the weight of your baby. You will feel much more renewed and refreshed after these kinds of gentle movements than if you were simply to collapse in a heap in front of the television. Remember to keep a large cushion handy beside you – for total relaxation after you have completed the stretches.

56 Side loosener

In these movements, the lower side of the trunk (the side that is lying against the floor) is gently stretched and the upper side is strongly contracted. You need to avoid overbalancing on to your back as you raise your upper leg, as this will reduce the contraction of the transverse abdominal muscles.

CAUTION
It is safe to lie on your back for the first 30 or so weeks of pregnancy, provided you feel comfortable. After this time, always recline or lie on your side for both stretching and relaxing. This avoids pressure on the main blood vessels to and from the uterus.

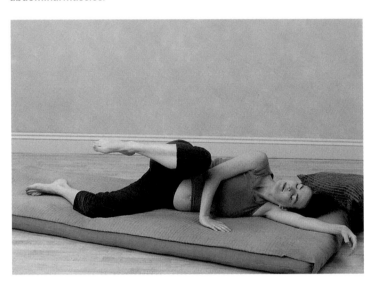

△ **1** Lie on your left side with your left knee bent (your other leg is more outstretched but still relaxed) and your left arm outstretched under your head. Place your right hand on the floor in front of you to help you maintain your balance. Lean forward as you raise your bent right knee and bring it toward your elbow.

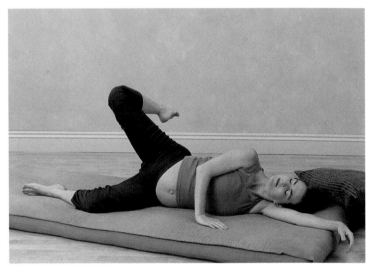

△ **2** Make gentle circles with the right knee, opening up your right groin and leg to extend your right leg slightly behind you. Do not over-stretch yourself. Return to your starting position with your right knee bent and repeat the circling movement. If you are skipping step 3, roll on to your right side and repeat with the left leg.

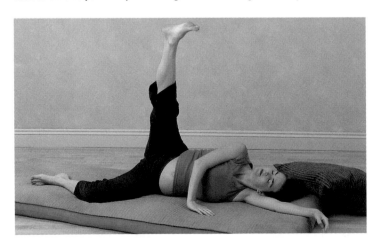

△ **3** This is an optional extra step. Only do this if it feels comfortable and enjoyable. If you have been circling the right leg, then stretch this leg straight up, with your ankle flexed, to open the right hip. Press forward into your right hand to avoid rolling backwards. Hold the stretch, feeling the muscles in your right side contract.

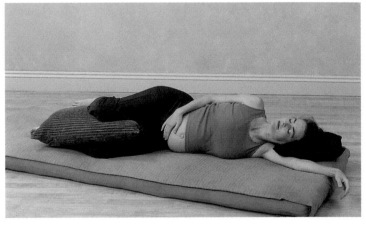

△ **4** At the end of a series of leg-stretches, relax for a few moments, placing the cushion between your knees to take the pressure off your lower abdomen.

57 Pelvic lift

In this position, you contract and strengthen the muscles around the base of your spine and make space at the front of your body. It is an excellent position for focusing on breathing deeply because you use all your abdominal muscles while the chest muscles are held open and immobile. It is also an excellent position for pulling your inner muscles in and up to strengthen the pelvic floor muscles in relation to the muscles of the abdomen and back.

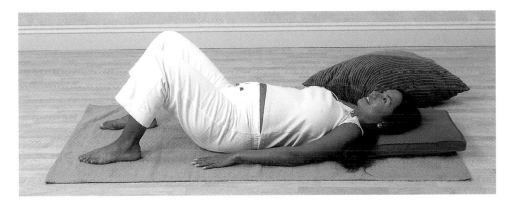

◁ **1** Lie on your back on the floor, with your head on a cushion if this feels more comfortable. Bend your knees and plant your feet on the floor more than hip-width apart. Turn your toes slightly inward to engage the muscles of the inner thighs and groin area. Place your arms alongside your body with the palms down. Now breathe in.

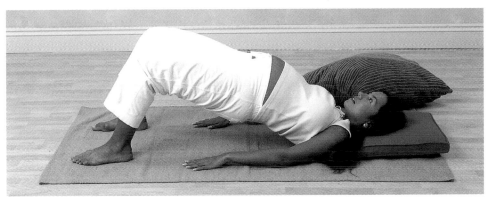

◁ **2** Breathe out as you lift your pelvis from the floor, engaging your perineal muscles and tucking your coccyx under to extend your lower back. Breathe in, continuing to lift your pelvis by contracting the muscles behind your waist and in your upper back. Breathe deeply in this position, focusing on your diaphragm muscle. Then lower your spine slowly to the floor, vertebra by vertebra from the neck downward. Rest and repeat several times.

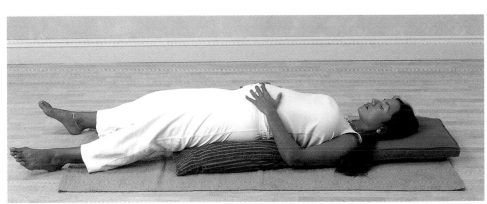

◁ **3** Lie on your back with a cushion under the small of your back. Stretch your legs out at least hip-width apart and place your hands around your baby. Close your eyes and relax deeply for a few minutes.

58 Double cycling

This isometric exercise strengthens the muscles in your feet, legs, hips and pelvis as you push your feet against those of your partner.

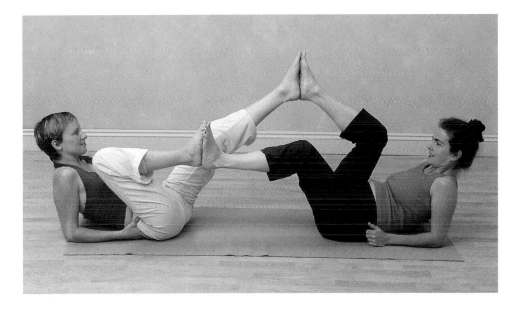

▷ Lie on your back on the floor, supporting your upper body on your elbows and forearms. Place your soles against your partner's soles and push against them as though riding a bicycle. For each person, one leg pushes forward against your partner as the other leg is being pushed back by your partner.

Changing positions in pregnancy

As the weight in your abdomen increases, it becomes more tiring to do certain everyday movements, such as rising from a chair or getting out of bed in the morning. This is inevitable, but there is no need to struggle if you learn some simple steps, preferably before you need them. As your baby grows in your womb (and also after the birth), you will be glad of your strong leg and arm muscles, as well as your strong back. Here's how to make these movements gracefully and easily.

59 Standing from sitting

It is more difficult to haul yourself out of a chair if you are slumped or sprawled backwards. Let your muscles hold your body firmly, so that gravity becomes your friend rather than your enemy. Of course, it is also easier to rise lightly from a firm, upright chair than a soft, low sofa, so choose carefully where you sit as well as how.

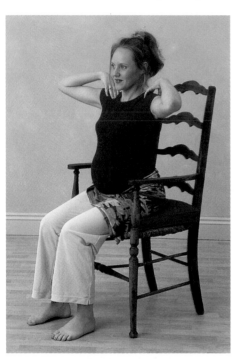

◁ **1** First sit up straight, so that your weight passes in a straight line from your head, through your neck and into your spine. Place your feet apart and firmly planted on the floor, ready to receive your weight. Raise your elbows to lift up through your spine and chest. Keep the stretch.

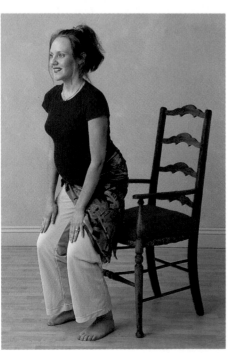

◁ **2** Lean forward with your back straight and place your hands on your thighs. The thighs are among the strongest muscles in your body, designed for weight-bearing, so use them fully to protect your lower back. Press hard on your thighs with your arms.

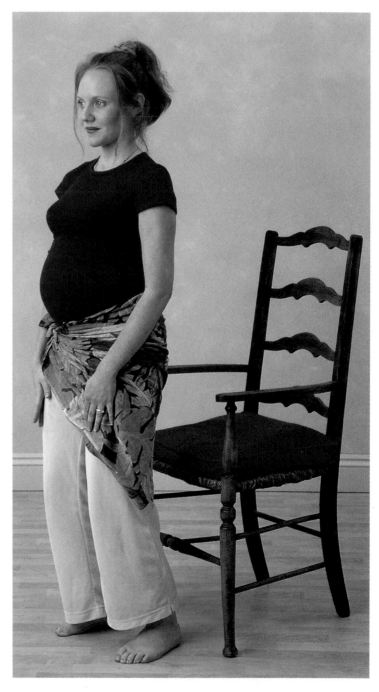

△ **3** Now rise gracefully and realign your spine before moving away from the chair.

60 Rolling out of bed

To begin this movement, make sure that you are lying facing the edge of the bed. You may like to rest or sleep with a cushion between your bent knees as this takes the pressure off your lower back and frees sensitive nerves in your back (particularly the sciatic nerve).

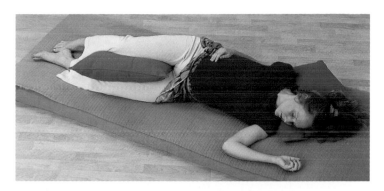

▷ **1** Lie on your side near the edge of the bed. You should have your lower elbow bent and your chest open – the ideal sleeping position for later pregnancy.

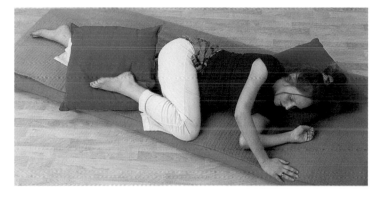

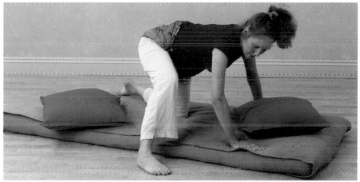

△ **2** To get up, roll more on to your front. Bring your top hand and your top knee over to the edge of the bed.

△ **3** Put your weight on your top hand, lifting your upper body, and slide your top leg over the edge of the bed to place your foot firmly on the floor. Raise your buttocks and rise out of bed.

61 Standing from lying

This technique will serve you well every time you get off your yoga mat after doing floor stretches or deep relaxation.

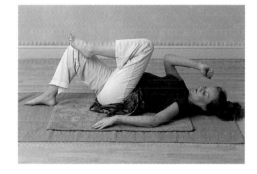

△ **1** Bend both knees and place your feet on the floor. Bring your right elbow to your left knee at about waist level.

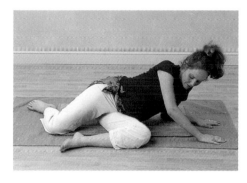

△ **2** Roll on to your left hip, leaning on your bent left leg, and support your upper body on your right hand. Bring the left hand up to shoulder level too.

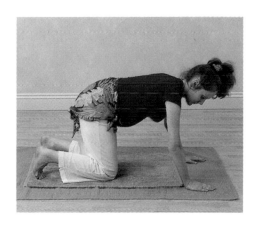

△ **3** Move on to all fours in the Cat Pose (45) and turn your toes under.

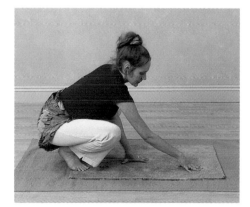

△ **4** Walk your hands back toward your knees. Your knees will then come up from the floor as your weight shifts back, so that you are in a squatting position, with your heels as low as possible.

▷ **5** Engage your thigh muscles and stand up slowly.

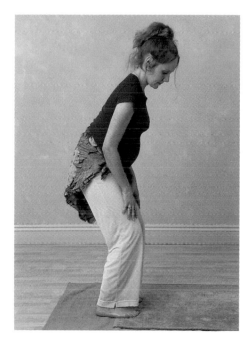

Some subtle yoga movements

Now for something totally different. You have discovered how effectively yoga helps you to strengthen your body and increase your awareness, and how you can use these benefits in your everyday life. Well, in yoga there are also certain positions that look – and are – simple to do, yet they create very subtle internal adjustments and strengthen groups of muscles that we are not usually aware of. These can bring huge benefits once you have explored, practised and become thoroughly familiar with them. These exercises require a calm, focused approach; in turn, they foster inner strength and self-confidence.

62 Gentle perineal stretch

This simple exercise should be done as often as possible from mid-pregnancy onwards, as it stretches all the muscles that make up the pelvic floor. It also strengthens, relaxes and brings awareness to the whole perineal area, which is the area through which your baby passes to be born. If the perineum is flexible, strong and lively, it helps you to give birth actively and with greater ease. You will be able to take your foot farther out to the side as you gradually loosen up with practice.

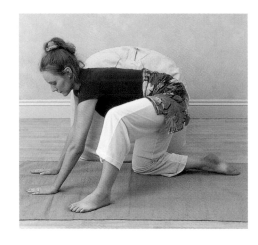

△ **1** From the Cat Pose (45), bring your left foot forward, placing it as far to the left of your hands as you can comfortably manage. Lean forward and breathe in deeply, keeping your spine stretched.

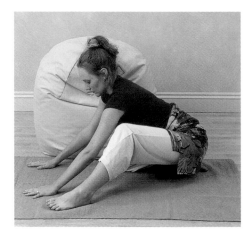

△ **2** Breathe out as you sit back on your right heel without moving your left foot. This stretches the perineal muscles. Repeat several times, then change sides and repeat.

63 Rib stretch with Namaste hand mudra

This powerful exercise helps you to open your lungs more fully and to breathe more deeply by stretching between the ribs, especially at the back where your ribs are attached to your spine. It brings increased awareness to your back and is also an isometric exercise that strengthens your arms and upper spinal muscles. A mudra is a gesture with a spiritual as well as a physical expression. Adding the Namaste Hand Mudra focuses your scattered thoughts and centres your vital energies. It should be practised frequently for greater posture awareness, increased vitality and a focused mind. In late pregnancy, this exercise helps to create more space in the chest for your lungs to expand as your baby develops below the diaphragm.

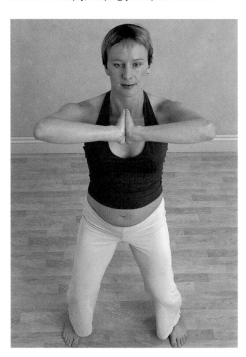

△ **1** Stand with your feet hip-width apart and knees loosely bent. Stretch the spine and drop the shoulders. Raise your elbows to the sides at shoulder height and press your palms hard together as you breathe in slowly and deeply. Feel your sternum rise and your ribs open at the back.

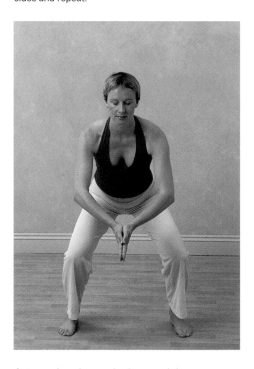

△ **2** Now, breathe out slowly as you bring your hands down, with palms still joined. Relax your chest completely. Pause and rest with the breath out, then repeat the sequence twice more. When you have finished, rest for a moment and observe how you feel deep inside.

64 Sectional breathing with mudras

You will probably be surprised to discover that your breathing changes according to the position of your hands in these subtle hand mudras. Ensure that the first three types of breathing come easily to you before you join them together in the complete yogic breath. Allow a minute or two of rest before and after this practice to gain maximum benefit.

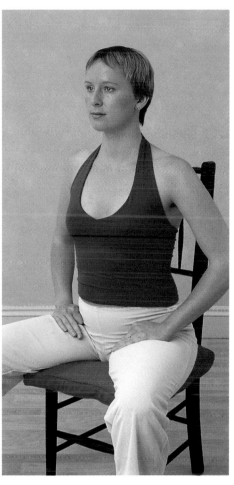

◁ **1** Sit up straight with your chest lifted to make room for your breathing muscles to move freely. Place your hands at your lower abdomen with fingers pointing toward each other. Join the tips of your index fingers and thumbs together to create a closed circuit of energy. Breathe in deeply and feel your abdomen expand as your diaphragm contracts downward. This is called "lower breathing" and gives you energy. Breathe out and repeat.

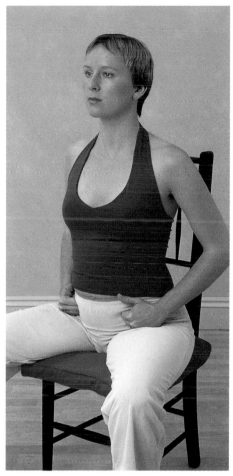

◁ **2** Now change your hand position, so that your fingers are curled into your palms and your thumbs are free. Breathe in deeply and feel your sternum lift and your ribs move out to the sides. This is called "middle breathing" and it also gives you energy. It comes to your rescue when your growing baby makes it difficult for your diaphragm to contract downward fully. Breathe out and repeat.

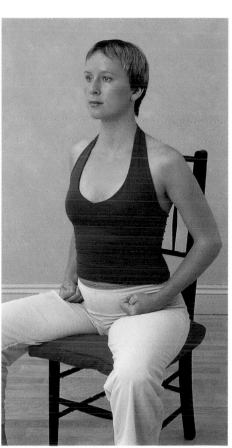

◁ **3** Change your hand position again, so that your thumbs are enclosed within your curled fingers. Breathe in deeply and feel how your upper chest is now moving much more freely. This is called "upper breathing" and is very useful if you have indigestion. Breathe out and repeat. You may also need this during labour, so start practising now.

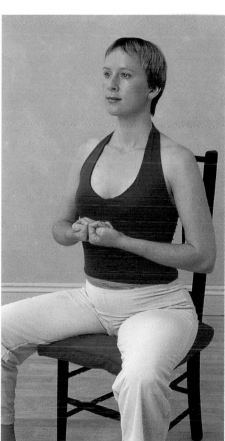

◁ **4** With your thumbs and fingers curled into your palms, press your knuckles together with the fingers of each hand back to back. Turn your palms upward, with your hands in front of you. Open your chest and breathe in fully, from the bottom of your lungs to the top. Breathe out fully and repeat several times. This is full yogic breathing, excellent for recharging your energy and integrating mind, body and spirit in the here and now.

balancing activity with relaxation

Our energy is called forth by stimulation, motivation, desire or need, which is the urge that gets us going every morning. Then we enjoy the experience of doing things and of being energetic, busy and involved. When this energy begins to ebb, we need to call it back within ourselves for recharging, so that we rest, relax and renew ourselves at every level by "just being".

If we are to maintain our zest for life, this cycle should be repeated throughout the day, until we finally wind down for our sleep at night. It is a rhythm as natural as breathing and it continues throughout life. Yet,

somehow, in our modern society, we have become addicted to just one phase of the cycle – the active phase – at the expense of the passive phase. We seem unable to respond to the need for rest even when we feel tired and depleted.

Yoga teaches us how to balance activity with rest, doing with being. It teaches us when and how to relax, and to respond to our body's signals that it is time for a short break. Deep relaxation does not take long and is less a question of time than of attitude. This vital life skill is one of yoga's most valuable gifts. First we become aware of the

rhythm of the breath and realize that each breath in is a muscular exertion; each breath out is the release that follows. Then we learn to apply this rhythm to all our activities – both mental and physical. We gradually learn to relax and release the toxins and tensions of living as they arise. It is their build-up that causes stress, congestion and poor functioning of body and mind.

With any relaxation practices, the most vital first step is to make yourself really comfortable, with support just where you need it, so that you can let all your muscles relax and your mind sink into repose.

65 Take your focus inward

"Time out" breaks work best when you have something gentle and non-stressful to focus on. Here are three useful suggestions.

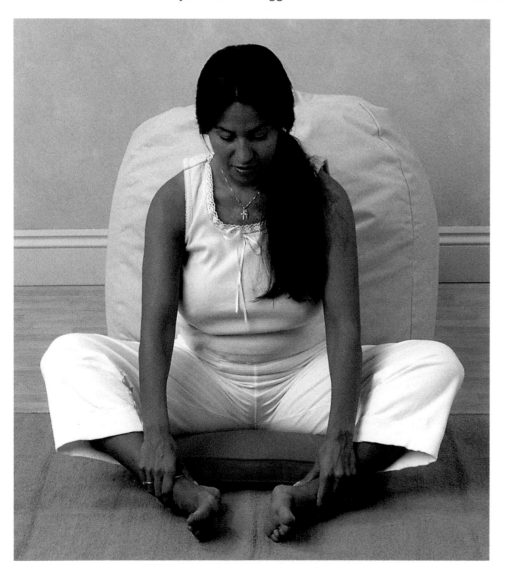

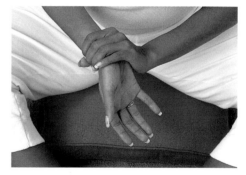

◁ **1** It can be very soothing to just sit quietly and turn inward, becoming aware of your growing baby. Try focusing on your own gentle breathing or on feeling your baby's life and movement inside you.

△ **2** Gently massaging your wrists and all the little joints in your hands releases tension and helps to balance the nervous system and pelvic area.

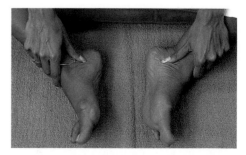

△ **3** The same principle applies to massaging your inner ankles. This is the reflex area for your womb and massaging gently helps tone and strengthen.

66 Focus on your baby

By now your baby is probably moving around vigorously, alternating between periods of sleep and activity, and growing into a real person. Get to know this person who is coming into your life. Enjoy the communication of loving touch between you.

67 Focus on yourself

Being pregnant, and focusing on your baby, does not make you any less of a person yourself. Relax for your own well-being, too.

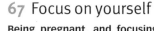
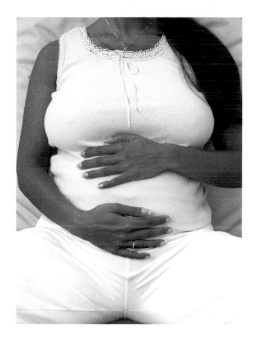

△ **1** Delight in noticing how your baby responds to the massaging movement of your loving hands.

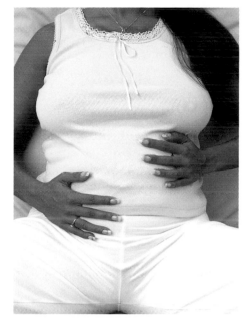

△ **2** Take time to explore your baby's contours. Are those heels? Is that a head?

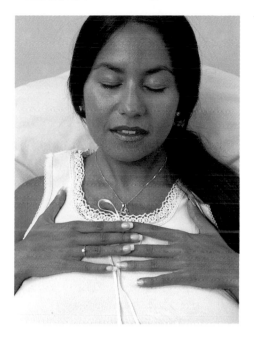

△ Feel your breathing and your own glowing heart centre radiating outward. Just be.

68 Relax with your partner

Both of you should celebrate the experience of your pregnancy. Invest time in getting to know this new person who is coming into your lives. Touch and talk to your baby together.

▷ **1** Relax while your partner explores your baby's movements. By placing his hand right under the base of your uterus (thumbs on pubis, fingers extended out toward the hip bones), he can give you a strong resistance that deepens your breathing while relaxing – excellent preparation for breathing through contractions without over-tensing muscles.

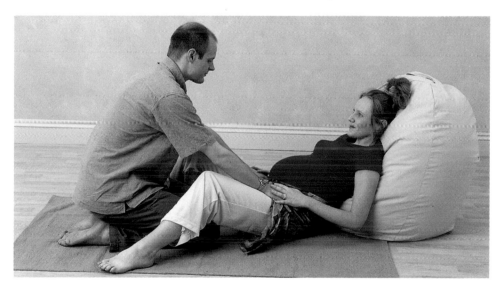

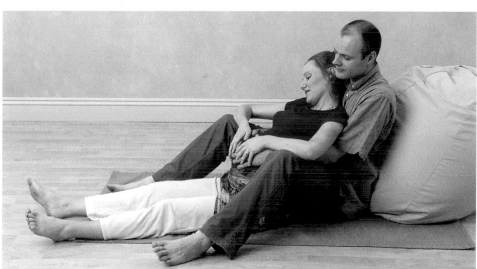

▷ **2** In joint relaxation with your partner, you can both place your hands on the baby. This quiet communication through touch generates harmony between the three of you – now and into the future.

deep relaxation

Deep relaxation is an essential part of your yoga practice. It may come at the end of a daily yoga exercise and breathing session, if you have time, or you may find it more convenient to divide your yoga session into two parts. You may like to practise yoga exercises with short rests for breathing and relaxation in the morning, then add an extra half-hour slot for breathing and deep relaxation at another time of the day when you will not be disturbed. The more regular your practice, the better the results.

69 Modified positions for deep relaxation

As your baby grows, lying on your back will no longer be comfortable and, as it can restrict circulation, it is not a good idea. The classical yoga relaxation position needs to be modified from about 30 weeks onwards. You can bend your knees or place a cushion or blankets under your hips, lie on your side or lean forward over a beanbag. You can even relax deeply while sitting up, as long as you are well supported and your legs are not hanging down. Below are six alternatives for you to try.

> **CAUTION**
> Those with high blood pressure should not rest with arms raised above their head – it makes the heart work harder. It is fine to raise arms while exercising, as the blood is already moving briskly.

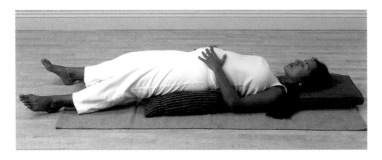

△ Place a firm cushion under the head, to lengthen the neck and stop the chin jutting up, and a soft one under waist and hips to ease the lower spine. With bent elbows, wrap your palms around the abdomen to keep contact with your baby.

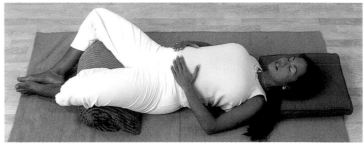

△ Bend your knees out to the sides and bring the soles of your feet together. Place plenty of soft padding under the thighs and knees. This makes more space in the lower abdomen for your baby.

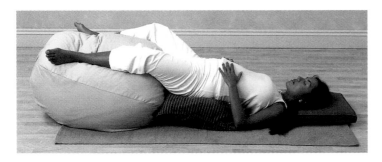

△ Place a beanbag under your legs and a cushion under the hips. Your raised legs improve blood flow to the heart and reduce swelling and aching in the legs; raised hips ease the lower back. This position also helps to turn a breech baby.

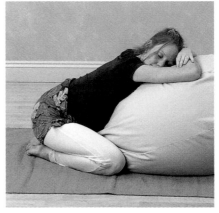

◁ Kneel down with knees wide, to allow plenty of room for your baby. Lean forward over a beanbag and rest your head in your arms. This is a very relaxing pose. The whole spine is gently stretched by the raised arms, the pelvis and hips are open, and the beanbag is taking the weight of the fetus.

▷ Push the beanbag against a wall for extra support and recline against it so that you are as comfortable as possible. Sit with your knees bent and out to the sides and add cushions underneath to open up your hips.

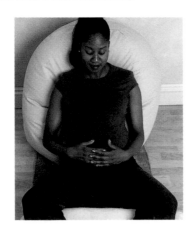

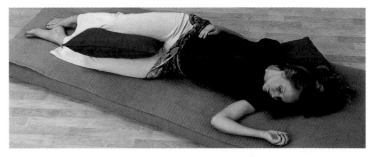

△ Lie on one side with a cushion between your knees and one under your head. Lying on your left side is a popular position as pregnancy advances, as it encourages the best presentation of the fetus for birth.

A sample mid-term practice

1

▷ **Swing and release** (42)

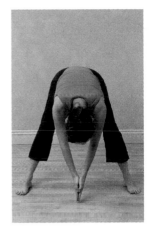

2

▽ **Supported pelvic floor lift** (51)

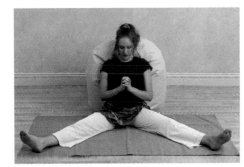

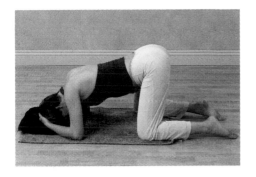

3

△ **Pelvic floor stretches** (50)

4

◁ **Sectional breathing with mudras** (64)

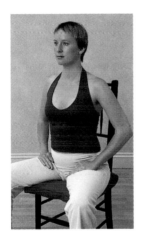

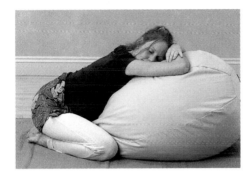

5

△ **Modified positions for deep relaxation** (69)

"The secret life stirs within me

O my darling, I can hear your

heartbeats ."

Indian birth song

Questions and answers

- **I get a lot of backache, especially in my lower back.**

This is usually because of tightness (caused by tension) in the muscles of the lower back as well as weakness in the lower abdominal and pelvic floor muscles. Practise the movements suggested in this chapter to strengthen these groups of muscles so that they can help to support your spine and keep your trunk in good alignment.

- **I get pain in my groin or pelvis, which seems to be caused by pressure or constriction.**

This can be due to muscular weakness or imbalance causing poor posture and undue pressure from the growing baby in the pelvic area. Practise abdominal strengthening, as well as upper spine and arm movements that lift your chest and pull the weight of your baby upwards. When resting, keep your legs up and your hips raised, to ease any pressure.

- **The pressure of the baby on my bladder wakes me up at night and I have to keep getting up.**

Avoid drinking at bedtime, and sleep on your side with a pillow between your knees to take the pressure off your bladder.

- **My joints feel so loose that I am afraid they will not support my increasing weight.**

Hormones are released during pregnancy that soften the ligaments that hold your joints in place. This is to prepare the pelvic area to open and let your baby pass through the birth canal. Avoid overstretching in any position, especially in those joints that bear the body's weight, namely your hips, pelvis, lower back and knees.

- **I can't get a really good night's sleep, and this is making me feel so tired all of the time.**

This lack of sleep can be due to all kinds of things – such as pressure on your bladder, indigestion, or swelling and puffiness in your legs. Exercises that will help to ease these conditions are given throughout this chapter. It may also help to play your relaxation tape in bed, just before you go to sleep. When you wake in the night, focus on your breathing, commune with your baby and repeat the "seed thoughts" and affirmations that we talked about in the introduction. Provided that your mind is profoundly relaxed and peaceful you should not be deprived of the rest that you need, even if you are not actually asleep.

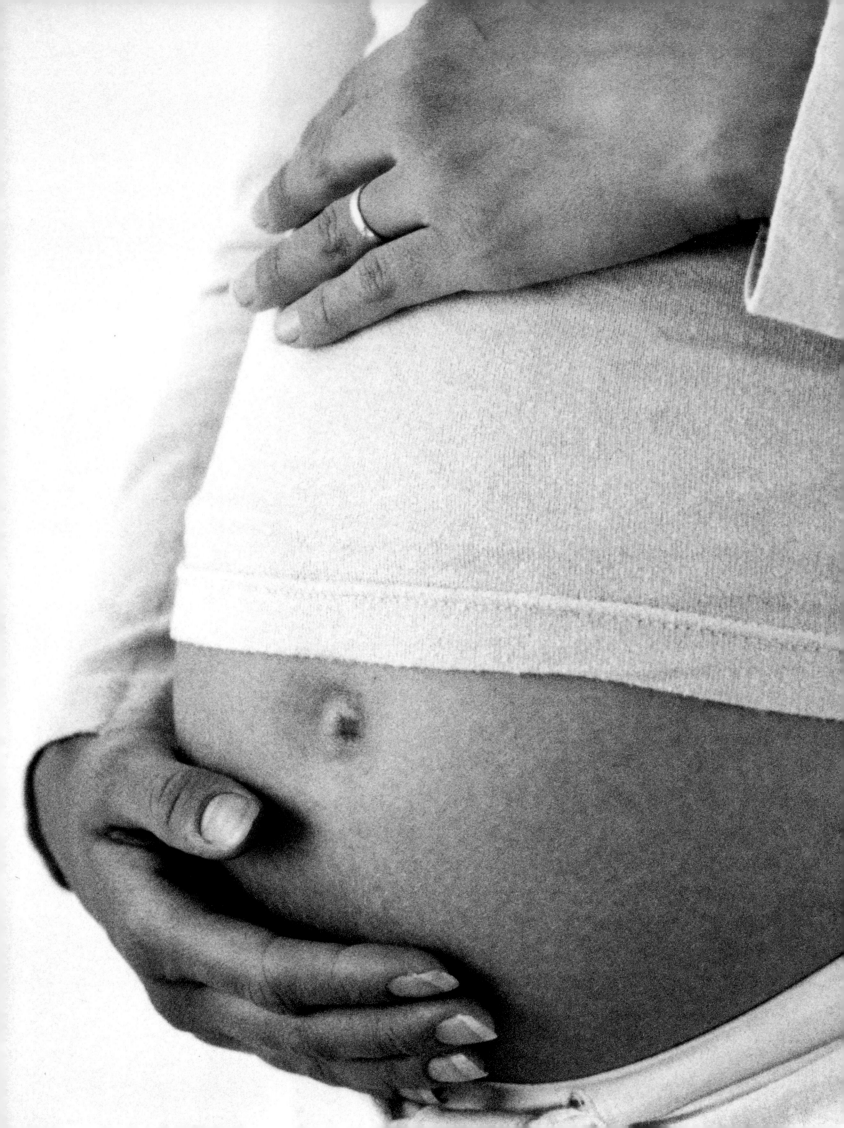

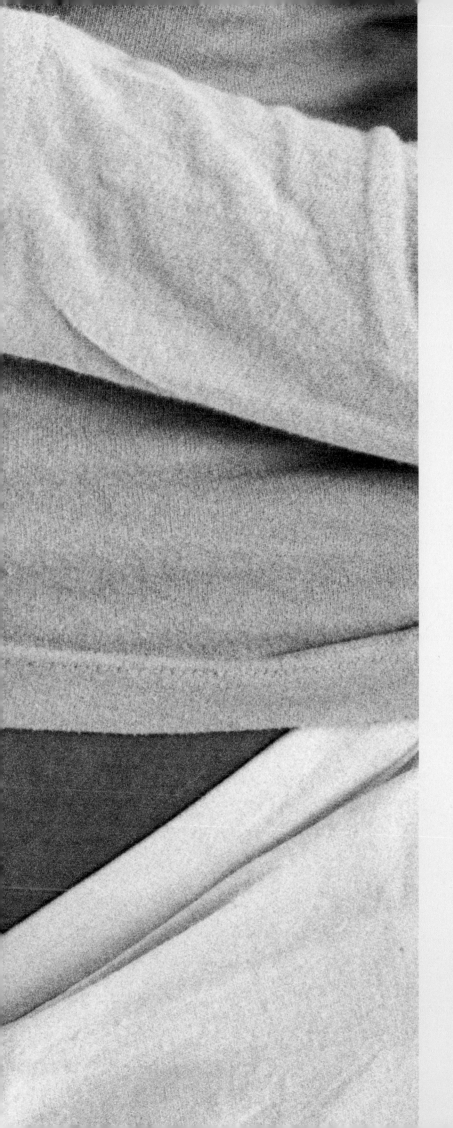

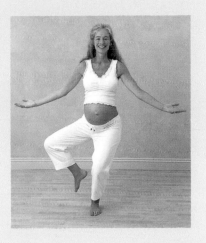

31+
weeks

During these last few weeks your priorities

will be to keep yourself as fit and comfortable

as possible, and to practise all the yoga

techniques that can help you during the

birthing process. These techniques prepare

you physically, mentally and spiritually for

labour, greatly empowering you from within.

However your birthing may unfold, yoga will

help you to feel centred and actively involved

with your birth.

Yoga in late pregnancy

Your baby will be growing rapidly by now, so your yogic priorities need to change. First, you will need to protect your back much more by ensuring that your pelvic and leg muscles are able to carry the extra weight properly. Your focus will be on building power in these supporting muscles. This means paying more attention to centring and grounding exercises, and always remembering to keep your knees well bent in any of the standing poses and movements. Cushions and beanbags should be used to support your back at all times, to enable you to rest more deeply during relaxation. Secondly, you will need to make more space for your baby, your breathing and your digestive organs. Finally, you will be focusing specifically on increasing the tone in your birthing muscles – in other words, the muscles of your lower back, abdominal area and pelvic floor.

70 Centring into the earth

This exercise combines both power and release. Imagine that you are hauling yourself up a ladder, one arm at a time, and then climbing down again as you support your weight with your arms. Your legs should be well bent to support your weight. Feel a line of strength developing along a vertical axis between earth and sky, passing through your body.

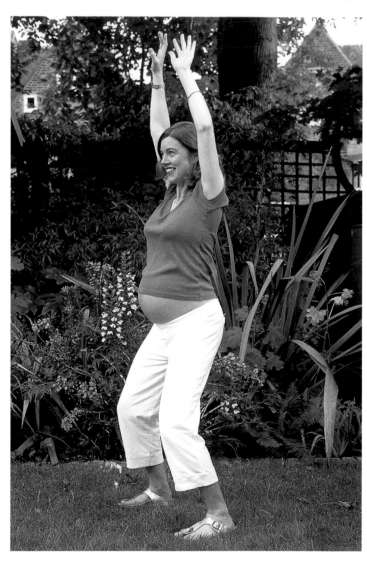

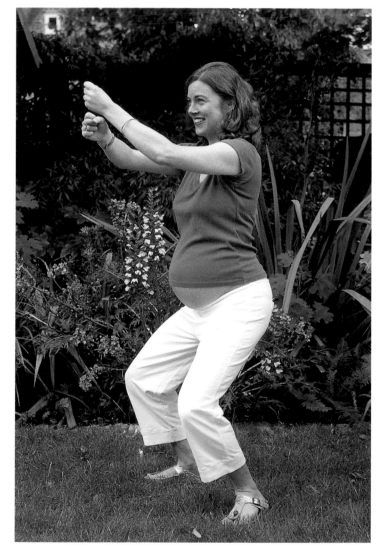

△ **1** You are going to climb up your metaphorical ladder. Stand with knees bent and spine loose. Now, stretch first one arm overhead and then the other, as though you were climbing a rope ladder without using your feet. Squeeze your fingers tightly to hold on to the ropes. When you get to the top, spend a few moments just hanging from both arms, alternately squeezing and releasing your hands.

△ **2** To climb down again, imagine you are going down a fireman's pole. All the strength is in your arms as you lower your weight one hand over the other down the pole. Slide down several times, bending your knees and grounding strongly along the vertical axis. These exercises can be done anytime, anywhere.

71 Supported side stretches

You need to practise side bending while sitting and resting your spine against a soft but firm support – here we show a beanbag placed against a wall, which is ideal.

▷ **1** Sit, leaning against a beanbag or a pile of cushions, with your legs stretched out in front of you and comfortably apart. Bring your hands behind your head with your elbows wide and pressed back to open your chest and stretch the sides of your body – you can breathe much more deeply in this position. Relax as you breathe and lengthen the breath out.

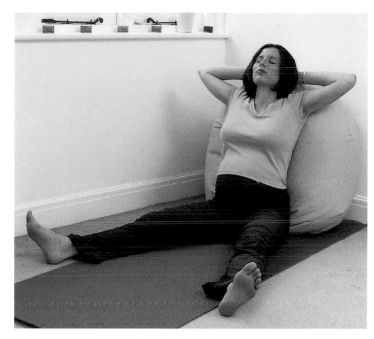

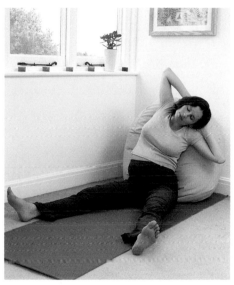

△ **2** Still leaning against the beanbag, tilt your upper trunk to one side as you breathe out. Breathe in to straighten up and then tilt to the other side as you breathe out again. Repeat a few times.

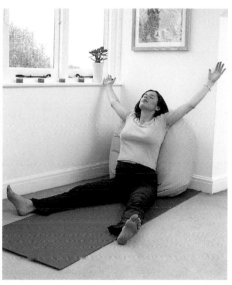

△ **3** Now, open your arms wide and stretch overhead, breathing deeply. This stretch really eases pressure in the lower body.

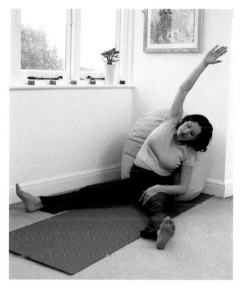

△ **4** Keep one arm overhead and take the other forearm on to your thigh for support, then tilt to the side on a breath out. Breathe in to straighten up and out to bend to the other side.

72 Hugging rest

This resting pose is ideal for late pregnancy. You may also find it comfortable for deep relaxation. The beanbag (or pile of cushions) supports your abdomen, spine and head. Spread your arms wide to lift and create more space in your chest.

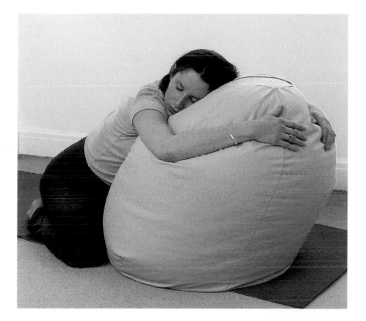

◁ Kneel down, facing the beanbag, with your knees spread wide to accommodate your baby. Now rest the front of your body and the side of your face against the softness of the beanbag and give it a big hug. Breathe deeply and relax completely.

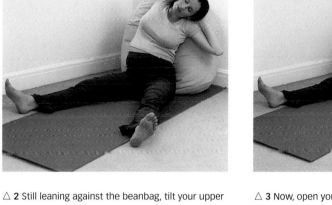
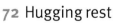

Light on your feet, $light$ at heart

To say that you are light and full of vitality may sound like a counsel of perfection when you are carrying around a baby that is almost ready to be born. It is, however, largely an attitude of both mind and heart. At this stage of your pregnancy it is very helpful to think "strong" and "graceful" simply to be in harmony with the pull of gravity and to lighten your spirits. Strong standing poses with graceful stretching movements will make sure that you stay full of joyful energy and in great shape.

73 Ball of energy (2)

This is a repeat of Ball of Energy (35), which was introduced earlier in your pregnancy. It is included here to remind you that it is a wonderful workout that lifts your spirits, and is just as useful for this late stage. Keep your legs strong and your knees well bent to protect your lower back as you stretch and bend your upper body in all directions.

CAUTION
Do only what you feel comfortable and happy with, at your own pace and without strain. Take plenty of rest between sequences.

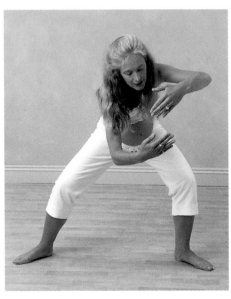

◁ **1** Take hold of your ball of energy in your hands. Take time to feel its weight and dimensions. Once you have its measure, start to play. Roll the ball between your hands, working your arms and shoulders.

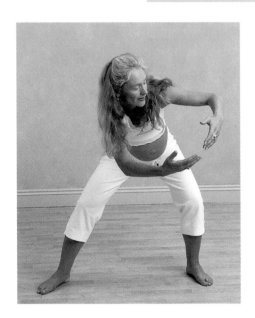

◁ **2** Now roll your imaginary ball out to one side, twisting in your upper body as you do so.

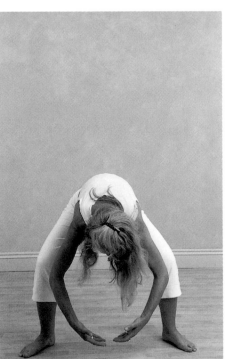

◁ **3** Bounce your ball on the floor, bending forward and relaxing your neck. Remember to keep your legs strong but relaxed and knees bent.

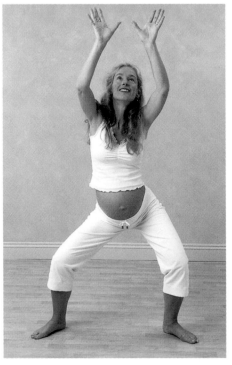

◁ **4** Toss the ball in the air, opening your chest and arching your upper back. Continue to improvise in whatever way you like – the idea is to be creative and have fun, as well as exercise your body.

74 Dynamic hip opener and stretch

This is a fluid, dancing movement, expressing feelings of well-being and exhuberance, lifting the spirits and opening the heart as well as lifting the upper body and opening the hips. It is excellent for creating lift in the upper body by stretching the arms up, which removes pressure around the diaphragm, and creating more space in the lower abdomen by opening up the hip joints.

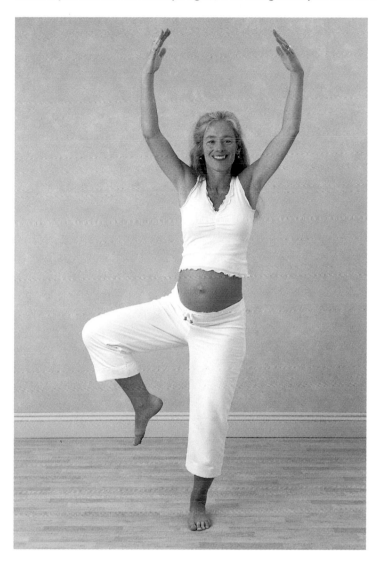

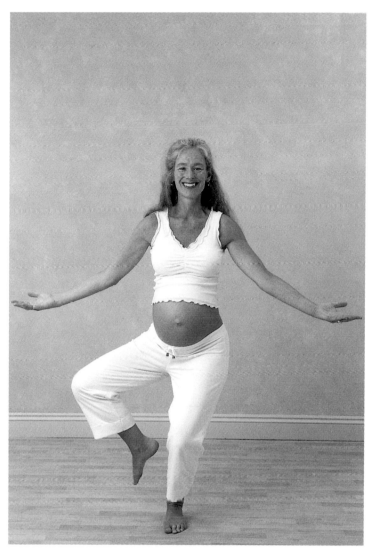

△ **1** As you breathe in, raise one leg to the side with the knee well bent and the hip open. At the same time, stretch up your arms and lift your sternum.

△ **2** As you breathe out, gracefully lower your arms and bent leg. Then begin again with the other leg. Repeat these two movements rhythmically, so that they merge into one fluid dance movement.

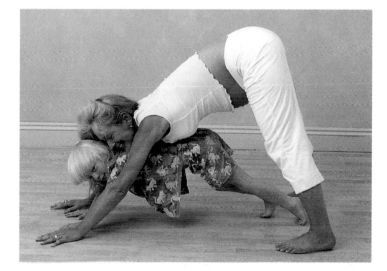

△ Sometimes you may need a little help to make your yoga more fun. Enjoy these unscheduled moments.

"Delight in yourself, in the meditative movement and the dance you are creating...this yoga is truly a dance..."

Janine Parvati Baker

Stretches for a $strong$ lower back and abdominal muscles

Think of yourself as an athlete in training who needs to build up power in specific groups of muscles for the task in hand, in this case giving birth. The muscles you will be using for childbirth are those in your lower back (for support and pushing against), your abdomen (to push the baby down the birth canal), your perineum and pelvic floor (for elasticity and control) and your breathing muscles (to make sure you stay energized throughout). You do not need complicated or expensive equipment in order to strengthen these particular muscle groups – you can find the props you need around your own home.

75 Kitchen yoga

Isometric exercises help to strengthen muscle groups and a good way to do this is to push or pull against an immovable object to create resistance. For these exercises, do make sure that what you are pushing and pulling against really is immovable.

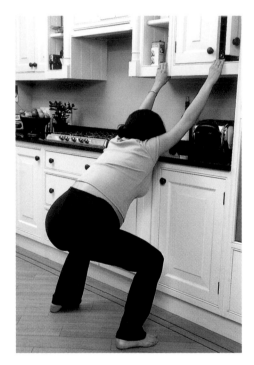

◁ **2** Bring your feet in line as you stand facing a ledge or shelf. Get a good grip with your fingers and, as you breathe out, pull down hard, bending your knees and sinking into a half squat. Hang there, breathing deeply and stretching through your trunk and arms as you work the muscles in your legs.

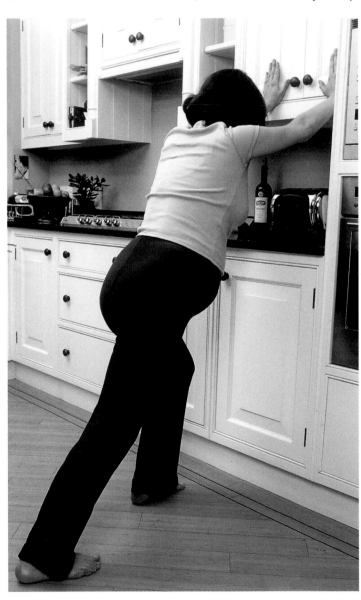

△ **1** Stand in front of a wall unit (or a wall). Place one foot well in front of the other, with the front knee well bent. Lean forward and place your palms on the unit at head height. Adjust your position so that you are the right distance away to push hard. Breathe in deeply and push, taking the force down through your back leg. Involve all your abdominal muscles on the breath out as you maintain the push. Swap legs and repeat.

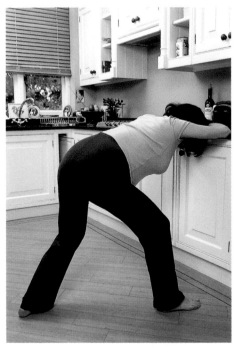

◁ **3** Stand in front of a counter top with one leg forward and the other back. Lean forward, bending your knees, and place your forearms on the edge of the counter with your forehead on top. Now, push down to open your chest and upper trunk, taking the push through your back heel as you lengthen your lower back. Hold, then repeat with the other leg back.

76 Stretch and squat with chair

Use a steady, upright chair to both stretch and squat down, as both positions will help to open up in the groin and stretch the pelvic floor. Keep your spine horizontal and your heels on the floor. To make the chair even steadier, push it against a wall.

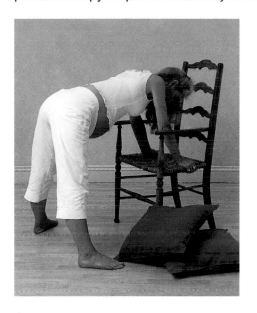

◁ **1** Stand in front of the chair with feet apart and toes turning outward, so that your knees will bend over your feet at the same angle. Bend forward and hold the sides of the chair seat, keeping your back stretched and horizontal.

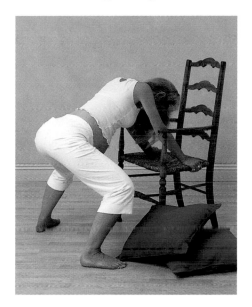

◁ **2** Squat down, bending your elbows to keep your back as flat as possible. Focus on stretching the inner thighs, the groin and the pelvic floor in preparation for giving birth. Breathe through this stretch, exhaling as you go down. Repeat frequently.

77 Perineal stretch with chair

Use a chair to help you when practising the Gentle Perineal Stretch (62) at this stage. For comfort, place a cushion under the shin and foot that you are going to sit on. This exercise will really help you to prepare your body for birthing. Finding the position in which your perineum is most relaxed and you can move your pelvic floor muscles easily is most important for this exercise – you might even get some kicks from your baby!

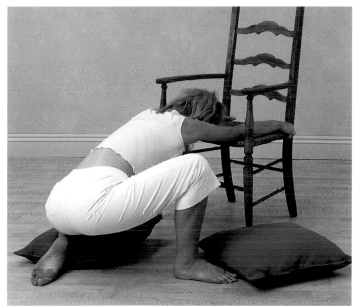

◁ Move from the Stretch and Squat with Chair (76) posture to a wide kneeling position, resting one knee on a cushion. Place the other foot out to the side of the chair. Now, holding on to the chair, press down and stretch through the whole perineal area on an out breath. Change legs and repeat the stretch. Practise frequently.

Relaxation throughout the day

Never miss an opportunity to relax, alone or in company. If you can relax the muscles that are carrying your baby at every opportunity, it will greatly enhance your feeling of fitness and well-being. Keep a beanbag handy for those blissful moments.

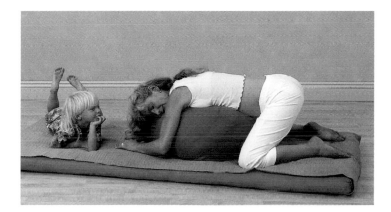

△ Kneel in front of a beanbag and flop over it to conduct weighty conversations with your toddler.

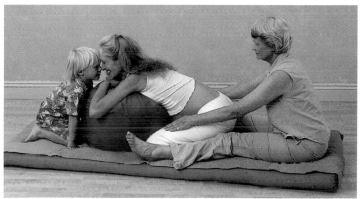

△ If someone can be gently massaging your thighs meanwhile, then so much the better. Relaxed enjoyment is the key.

Yoga movements for tone and energy

All these standing and walking movements help to create space in your abdomen and between your hips so that your baby has more opportunity to move around and get settled in a good position ready for the journey down the birth canal. So wriggle around as much as you can! In addition, shifting your weight from one leg to another, either in standing or walking poses, helps to prevent or ease varicose veins and swelling caused by an uneven distribution of your body weight.

78 Upper torso circles

These stretches lift your chest up and away from your abdomen, relieving pressure on your abdominal organs and giving your baby more room to change position. They help to diminish the effects of wind or gas in your digestive system and alleviate heartburn in the last few weeks of your pregnancy.

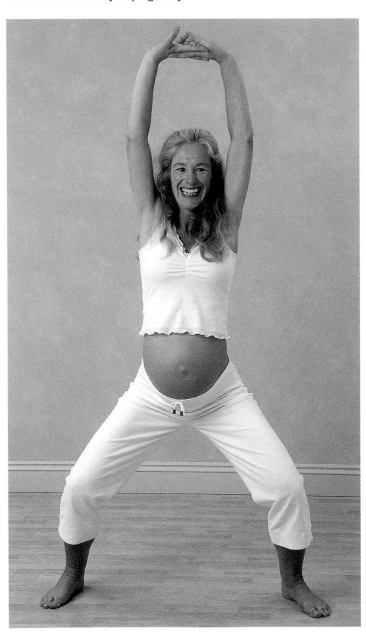

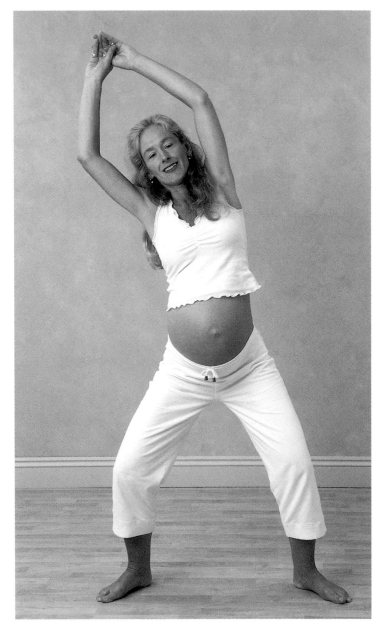

△ **1** Stand with feet wide and knees well bent. Stretch your arms overhead with hands clasped and palms facing the ceiling. Breathe in and stretch up some more.

△ **2** Make large clockwise circles with your clasped hands as though you were swinging a rope around above your head. After some clockwise circles, repeat the movements anti-clockwise. Engage the muscles at the sides of your body as you circle your upper torso and shoulders.

79 Pink panther strides

These exaggerated strides open the hips and pelvis, as well as the chest for deeper breathing. They work the muscles at the sides of the abdomen and spine. You will have to concentrate to make sure that you use the right combination of legs and arms at the right time.

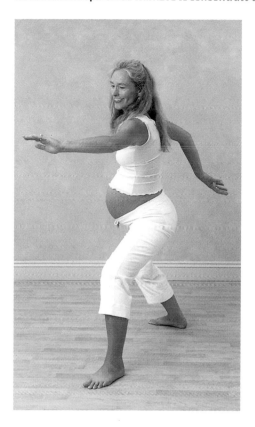

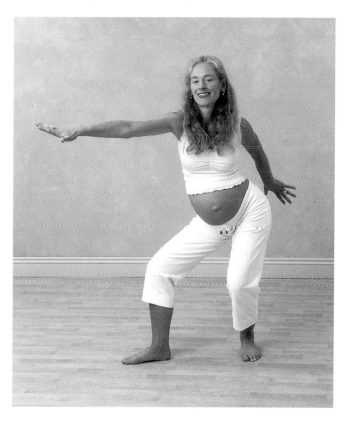

◁ **1** Start off in a centred, firmly based standing pose with feet together. Now stride forward boldly with your left leg, swing your left arm forward and your right arm back. Freeze in this position.

▷**2** Making a big stride, bring your right foot forward along with your right arm, taking your left arm back. Holding in between, repeat these alternating strides. Now change to left leg forward, right arm forward and right leg forward, left arm forward, and repeat for a few strides. Then swap over again to left-left and so on.

80 Hip drops

This is another name for the famous "Charlie Chaplin walk". Hip Drops can be practised either standing on one spot or striding forward. This walk will ease pressure in your hips, pelvis and lower back and encourage your baby to join in and get moving. Try to get the rhythm of "strong then limp" in each hip as you wobble forward in an aimless sort of way with a silly grin on your face. This isn't as odd as it sounds – a tight jaw can be a sign of a tight pelvis. Your midwife may even ask you to drop your lower jaw during labour to relax your pelvis.

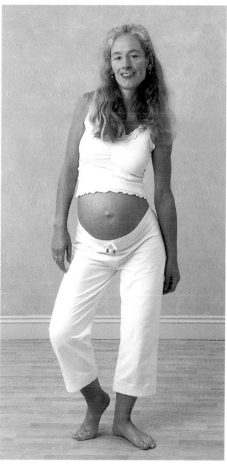

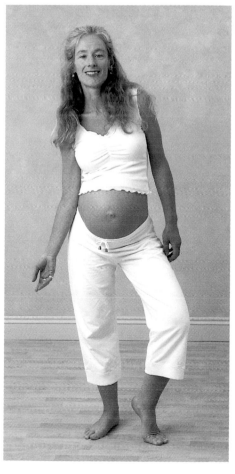

△ **1** Turn your feet out. Stand on your left foot with left leg strong. Drop your right hip, letting your right leg dangle loosely. Swing your limp right leg forward.

△ **2** Stand on your right foot with right leg strong, dropping your left hip and letting your left leg dangle loosely. Repeat.

Helping your baby move into position

You will find that your baby is sensitive to your moods, shares your enjoyment and joins in with all your activities. So the more that you dance around and stretch, and open and tone your body, the better he, she or they will like it. Your centre of gravity lies deep within your pelvis. The opening up of your hips and pelvic area, plus all the activity, will encourage your baby to find the very best position to be in as birth approaches. Putting aside time each day for a few minutes of energetic yoga dance, followed by perineal breathing, is the perfect way to prepare for labour with your baby. Don't forget that all these rotating, twisting and opening movements of the hips should be done with knees bent.

81 Knee circles

This is a balancing exercise that shakes out your hips and legs as you get into a knee-swinging stride. It is a loosening and strengthening movement, good for the circulation and for lifting your mood. If you feel wary about trusting your balance, place one hand against a wall for support. These knee circles should be done smoothly and lightly. Keep arms, shoulders and neck relaxed. The raised leg is also kept as loose as possible throughout.

▷ **1** Stand on your right leg, with arms spread to the sides at shoulder level for balance and your spine erect. Now swing your left knee up in front of you as high as is comfortable.

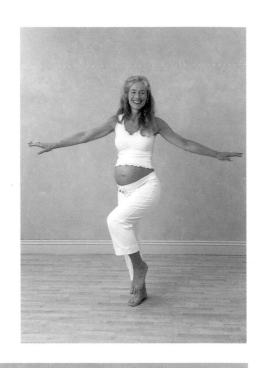

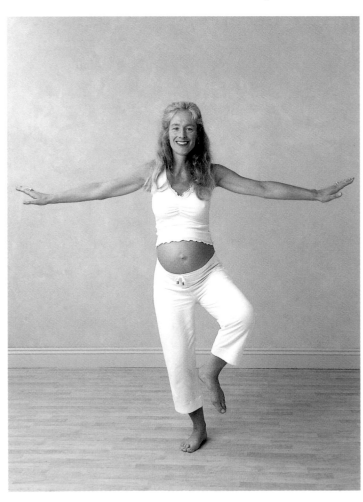

△ **2** Bring your left knee to the side to open your left hip and so make more room in the abdomen and pelvis.

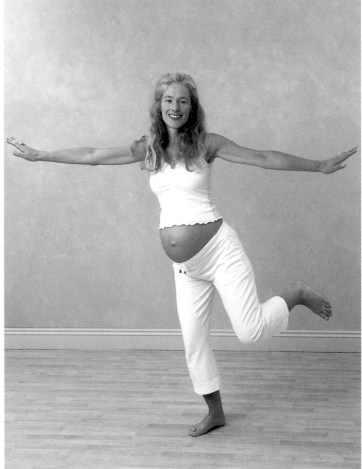

△ **3** Now, swing it round behind you and kick back strongly with your left foot. Finally, swing your knee forward, straightening your left leg and placing your left foot firmly on the floor. Repeat with the right knee.

82 Pushing the sky

In this pose you are pushing your palms against nothing. The aim is to lift and strengthen your upper body and make space in your lower body as you flex your thigh muscles. It is an empowering position. Use your diaphragm and breathe deeply, involving all your abdominal muscles. This pose helps prevent or repair a split in the central band of abdominal muscles, particularly if you are expecting twins.

▷ **1** Stand with feet wide and toes pointing outward so that you can bend your knees deeply and hold this position. Keep your spine erect and raise your arms overhead. Now push upward even further with first one palm and then the other, turning your palm upward if you can and lengthening through each side of your body in turn.

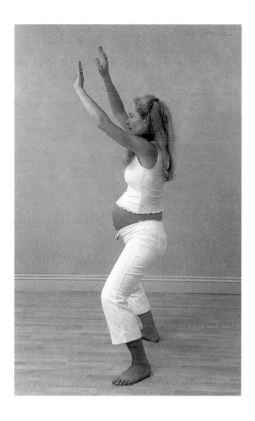

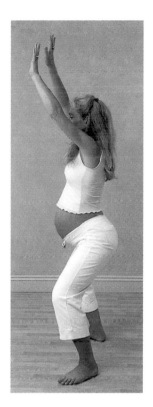

◁ **2** Keep your arms directly overhead. Push upward while going into a semi-squat downward, lengthening through your middle on an out breath.

83 Standing twist

This is a good position either on its own, to ease tension in the neck and shoulders, or as a counter-pose to the strong sideways stretch of the Knee Circles (81). Breathe deeply and twist through the whole torso.

84 Seated perineal stretch

Now that your baby has grown so much, a low stool and several cushions are useful props for this modified version of the Gentle Perineal Stretch (62). Place one cushion on the stool and the others under your dropped knee as required. Remember throughout that it is the breathing that creates all of the action when you are stretching the yogic way – otherwise nothing happens, or you simply stretch a little in the groin area.

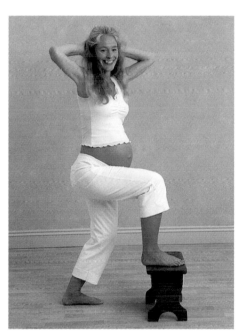

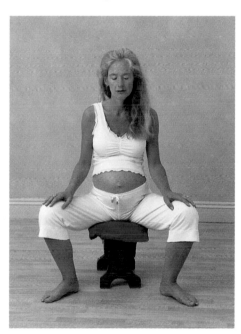

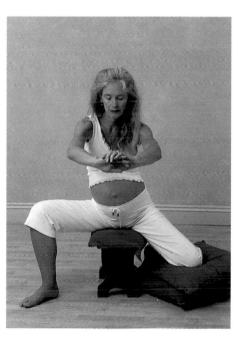

△ Place your right foot on a low stool or chair, making sure that your thigh is parallel to the floor. Raise your arms and open your elbows so that your chest feels open. Place your palms behind your head with neck strong and straight. Breathe in. As you breathe out, twist your head and shoulders to the right. Your upper chest will follow, but your lower body is kept steady by the bent leg. Repeat the twist to the left, with your left foot on the stool.

△ **1** Sit on a cushion astride a low stool, with your knees wide and feet firmly planted on the floor in front. Stretch up through your spine by pressing your palms against your spread thighs.

△ **2** Pressing down firmly into your right foot, drop your left knee back and down on to the pile of waiting cushions, to stretch through the left groin and the perineum. Clasp your hands, breathing in as you push the palms away from you in a forward stretch, taking your weight through your strong right leg. Stretch further as you breathe out and lift through the spine as you breathe in several times. Change legs and repeat.

Preparing for labour with kneeling poses

Sitting on your heels, with a cushion between your buttocks and your heels for comfort, is one of the best positions you can adopt at this stage of pregnancy. Your spine is erect, with the coccyx hanging freely, and the trunk's weight is flowing down naturally through your legs and into the floor. This open position means that your baby's head has the maximum amount of space in your pelvis. With the padding from the cushions, you can comfortably maintain this position while you are doing other things, such as chatting to a friend. Kneeling poses also prepare you for a birthing position on all fours – a comfortable and popular choice.

85 Chest openers

Clasping your hands behind your back can be difficult for some people, yet it is well worth persevering because it is a good way to open the shoulders and chest, straighten the upper spine and make more space – especially to ensure a better position on all fours.

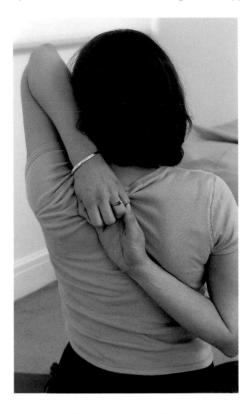

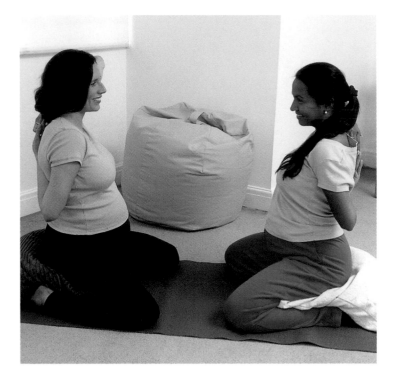

◁ **1** This is the classical position. One elbow is brought up to ear level and then bent to bring your palm against your upper back, while the other elbow is brought down by your side and bent to bring the back of your hand against your upper back. The two hands find each other (sometimes with help from a friend) and are clasped. They pull on each other to create the stretch at the front of the body.

△ **2** Take a few deep breaths in the position, then relax.

▷ Here is another chest opener with variations for different levels of suppleness in the shoulder joints. Take both arms behind you. For an easy version, hold each elbow with the opposite hands. For a stronger stretch, press your palms together behind your shoulder blades in the Namaste (prayer) position. Lean forward to stretch the spine at the back, making room between your knees for your baby. If leaning far forward is uncomfortable, then just lean a little way, or lean on to a low bed – whatever you are happy with.

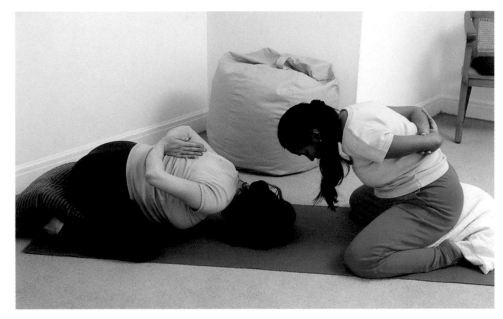

86 Tiger stretch and relax (2)

Do you remember Tiger Stretch and Relax (1) (48)? It is important to carry on with this stretch in the final few weeks of your pregnancy, as it is an excellent way to revive the circulation in your legs as your growing baby presses upon the major arteries, veins and nerves in the lower back and groin. Alternate this exercise with the Active Kneeling Stretch (87) that is shown below.

▷ Begin in the Cat Pose (45). Stretch your right leg out behind you, parallel to the floor. Let it drop and trail out behind you, dropping your right hip. Shake it to relieve stiffness after kneeling or sitting. Readjust your position and do the same with the left leg.

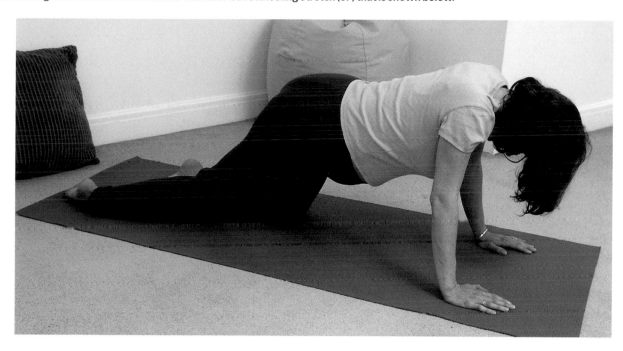

87 Active kneeling stretch

Another good kneeling stretch for the final weeks of pregnancy. Alternate with the Tiger Stretch and Relax 2 (86).

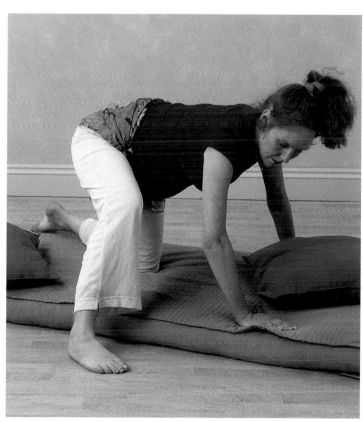

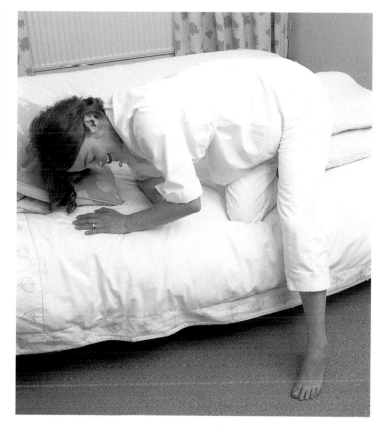

△ **1** From a kneeling position, put your weight on both hands, lifting your upper body, and slide your right leg over to place your right foot firmly on the floor. Now raise your buttocks on an in breath and stretch your lower back as much as possible as you flex your bent right knee and open your right hip joint. Keep your weight equally distributed on your left knee, your right foot and your hands, using a gentle rocking movement. Repeat on the other side.

△ **2** This is a gentler version of the active kneeling stretch, using a bed, as you may not feel strong or supple enough to kneel on the floor comfortably as birth approaches or during labour. Kneel on a low bed, resting on your forearms, and let one leg drop toward the floor at the side of the bed. Breathe deeply, focusing awareness on your lower back. Repeat on the other side of the bed.

Massage, breathing and relaxation

These last few weeks are the time to take full advantage of all the help and support that family and friends can give you. You need to build up your reserves of physical and emotional strength in preparation for the birth, and the changes in your life once your baby is born. So rest and rest again, at odd moments and in whatever position you find comfortable. While relaxing, breathe deeply in order to nourish both your baby and yourself, and to let go of aches and tensions. Massage can be a great help, and the person doing it does not need to be an expert, as long as they are happy to do what you ask.

▷ **Cuddles and closeness are especially soothing and sustaining during this final period of waiting. Let the whole family join in.**

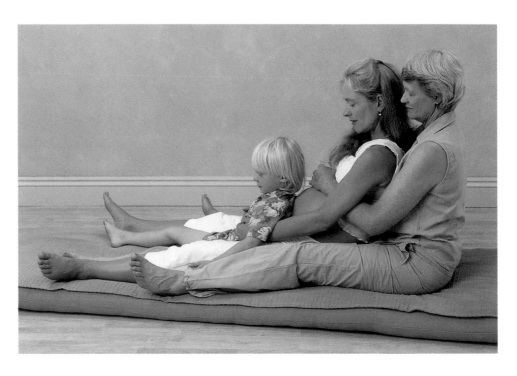

88 Back massage for deep breathing

This is one of the most soothing things that one friend (or partner) can do for another. It can be heaven for the recipient and also very soothing and relaxing for the person doing the massage. The recipient kneels with her knees wide and toes touching, and stretches over the beanbag in a relaxed and comfortable position. The beanbag will yield to fit the baby comfortably. The masseuse can kneel comfortably to one side, leaning forward slightly to massage her friend's back in soothing, circular movements. Both of you should make sure you are relaxed and comfortable before starting the massage. If pregnant herself, the masseuse should not lean forward too far, as this could cause backache.

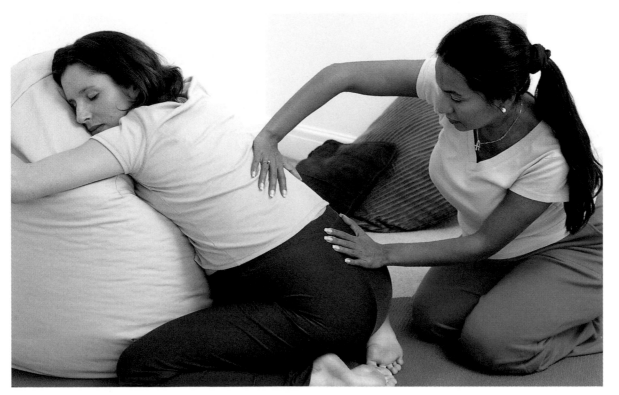

◁ The masseuse lays both hands gently on the recipient's back and leaves them there for a moment. This establishes a gentle contact while she co-ordinates her breathing with that of the recipient. "Two breathing as one" is a key feature in massage. The masseuse then moves her hands as the recipient is breathing out (and therefore relaxing), lifting them slightly to allow the recipient room to breathe in deeply into her back lungs beneath the helper's hands. See exercise 49 for back massage guidelines.

89 Ankle massage in supported Warrior pose

The purpose of this exercise is to relax the thigh and calf muscles passively while a friend supports your stance and massages your lower leg. Leaning against a wall with your head on your hands lifts your upper torso and creates more space for you to breathe deeply into your abdominal, pelvic floor and buttock muscles. You will find that this brings blissful relief generally, and relieves tight calves and lower backache in particular. Cramping in the calf muscles is common in late pregnancy as your legs cope with the extra weight and your blood circulation slows down.

▷ **1** Stand tall and lean your head against a wall with your forearms at head height. Take one foot forward. Bend the front knee and stretch through the back leg, as you take your weight into your back heel. Your friend should now get into a stable position where it is easy and comfortable for them to massage your leg.

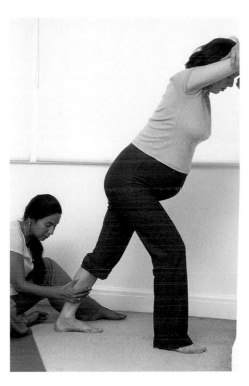

▷ **2** Your friend should hold the ankle of your back leg to ensure that it doesn't lift from the floor as you lean forward. This increases the stretch in the calf. Lean into the stretch as you breathe deeply.

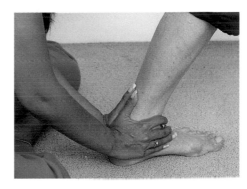

▷ **3** Your friend can now slowly massage your lower leg, breathing in time with your own breathing, to release stiffness and tension and improve blood circulation.

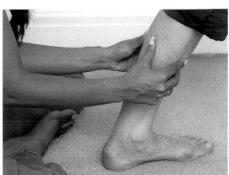

90 Supported reclining

Lying on your back after about 31 weeks is neither comfortable nor recommended, as the weight of your baby can put pressure on the vena cava, which carries blood from the uterus to your heart. Instead, recline at a comfortable angle on a nest of cushions, either on your bed, sofa or the floor. Have your "nest" ready and waiting for you, so that whenever you get the chance you can crawl in, lie back, close your eyes and relax.

▷ **1** Lean back against a beanbag or pile of cushions. Make sure that your trunk is raised and your head is at a comfortable angle. Add cushions under your bent knees to lessen the pressure in your lumbar area.

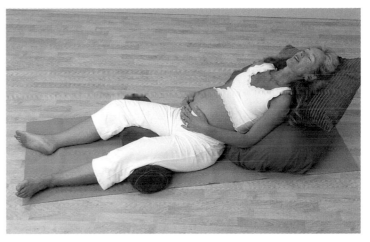

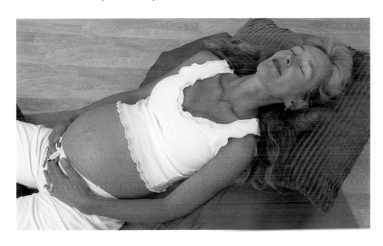

△ **2** You can place your hands over your baby to increase your loving connection to him or her – or them.

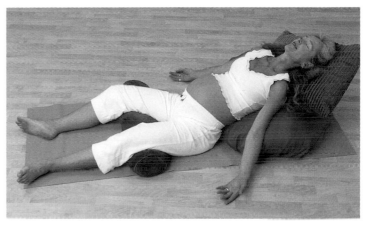

△ **3** If you prefer, let your hands simply flop to the sides. Breathe deeply and feel yourself letting go of any strains or tension.

Preparing for birth through massage

Self-massage is a technique that pays great dividends in terms of ease during the birth and afterwards, as breastfeeding is being established. It is easy and relaxing to do, and well worth spending some time on. You do not need to use any oil for your massage, but if you wish to, then use pure plain oils as some oils are not recommended during pregnancy – check with an expert aromatherapist first. There are five main areas to focus on.

1 The base of the body, the perineum, has to be strong to support the contents of the abdomen, especially as your baby grows much heavier in later pregnancy. At the same time, however, it will also have to yield and stretch in order to let your baby pass down the birth canal. Nature provides for this change in texture by releasing "loosening" hormones that soften the ligaments. You can also help to improve elasticity in this area by self-massage. Massaging the yogic way can greatly increase the comfort and ease with which you give birth, and possibly prevent a tear or the need for a surgical cut (episiotomy).

2 Up to 36 weeks into your pregnancy, your breasts can be prepared for breast-feeding by regular massage. In Western societies, women's breasts are always covered up and so become unnaturally soft. Massage helps to tone and strengthen the breasts and make the surrounding areola more elastic.

3 The abdomen has to stretch a great deal during pregnancy and can be made much more elastic by regular massage. This also helps to prevent stretch marks.

4 Your feet and ankles may be swollen by fluid retention. Massage can often help to relieve this congestion, thus easing pressure and swelling and the resultant aches and pains.

5 While you have the massage oil on your hands, don't forget your face. Gentle circular movements over the face relieve tiredness and tension and feel soothing and relaxing.

how to massage yourself

You may like to take a relaxing bath first or just apply a hot, wet flannel to the area to be massaged. The hot flannel brings the blood

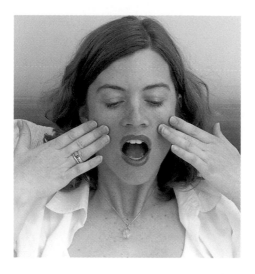

△ **Massaging the muscles around your mouth is helpful for keeping your lower jaw dropped and your face generally relaxed during labour.**

closer to the surface, which is soothing in itself. Settle yourself with the oil, if using, beside you. Find a comfortable, supported position. Reclining is probably best, either against a beanbag or on your bed.

Apply a little oil, if used, to your hands. Your touch should be exploratory but relaxed and gentle, indeed almost passive and reflective. Use your breathing actively as part of the massage. The stretching of tight skin and tissues is not caused by your fingers but by the relaxation of the tissues against your fingers when you breathe out. So, whatever part you are massaging, work with awareness of your breathing, moving your fingers on the out breath.

▷ **Massage your breasts with gentle strokes, going toward the areolas. Do not massage the nipple area itself (see the Caution box) and avoid any breast massage after about 36 weeks.**

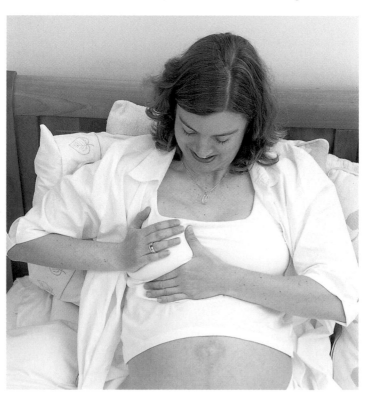

CAUTION
Nipple massage: Do not massage the nipples themselves. However, if you have reached your due date, then tweaking your nipples gently between thumbs and index fingers can be an effective way of stimulating producton of the hormone oxytocin and so helping to bring on labour.
Perineal and vaginal massage: Never pull or attempt to stretch these tissues manually.

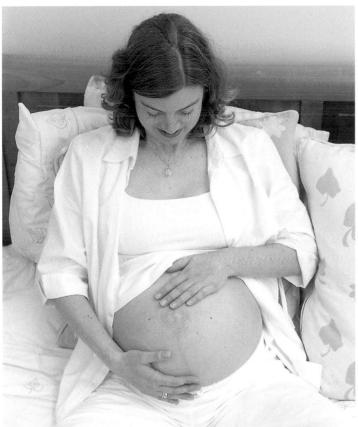

"From early days,

Beginning not long after that first time

In which, a Babe, by intercourse of touch

I held mute dialogues with my Mother's heart..."

William Wordsworth

◁ **Very gentle abdominal massage helps to prevent stretch marks.**

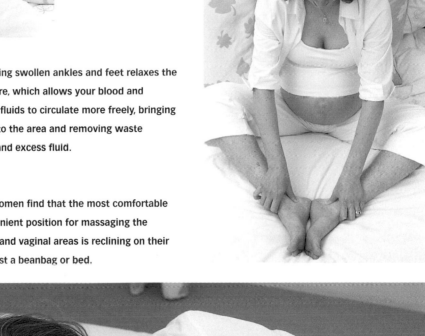

perineal massage

It is truly amazing just how quickly the normally tight tissues in the perineum, vagina and abdomen will stretch with regular massage. The more that you are able to pre-stretch these tissues before the birth the better you will return to your original shape after it. Start around 36 weeks and practise once a day.

Use a light touch to explore the layers of tissues along the back wall of your vagina and the skin that separates your vagina and anus. It is this area that will be most stretched during the birth of your baby and is most prone to tearing.

Insert two fingers into the vagina up to the first knuckle, progressing to the second knuckle with practice. Press against the back wall of the vagina, against the spine, while breathing deeply. Feel the muscles under your fingers as they engage on the breath out. As space is created, move in further and exert a little more pressure. Using your breath in this way is like blowing up a balloon. Nothing much seems to happen at first, but soon your perineal tissue starts to give and then begins to stretch. You will be amazed how much you can stretch it, simply by breathing out into the areas under your fingers.

▷ **Massaging swollen ankles and feet relaxes the tissues here, which allows your blood and lymphatic fluids to circulate more freely, bringing nutrients to the area and removing waste products and excess fluid.**

▽ **Most women find that the most comfortable and convenient position for massaging the perineum and vaginal areas is reclining on their side against a beanbag or bed.**

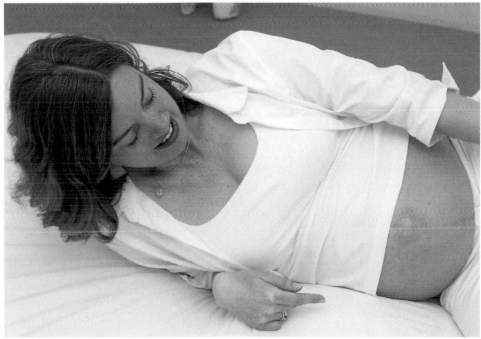

Yoga for labour and birthing

Day by day, your baby is getting ready to be born. Your body responds to your baby's signals with practice contractions of your womb and the release of birth hormones. This is a time of great excitement and some uncertainty, of exhilaration and suspense. You need yoga more than ever, to create and maintain feelings of peace and surrender in preparation for your baby's journey into the world. All your stretching and breathing practices will come into play during labour and the birth itself.

the labour circuit

Each birth is unique and each labour starts differently. As you approach your due date, it can be helpful to choose and practise several positions to use during early labour. These should keep you comfortable and help you to breathe through your contractions, making them as effective as possible. These positions make up your "labour circuit". The labour circuit allows you to stay in your own unique rhythm and to ease the descent of your baby by making full use of gravity. If all goes well, it may help you right up to the point where you are fully dilated. Every 15–20 minutes, move from one position to another position around your circuit. You will find that one or two positions will begin to feel the most comfortable and secure and you will tend to stick with those.

From time to time, also use movements 79 (Pink Panther Strides) and 80 (Hip Drops). These will loosen up your hips and back and release tension. Alternating positions is particularly helpful if labour is slow to get established, as this helps the baby's head to press down on to the cervix. What follows are some suggested positions for inclusion in your own labour circuit.

> **CAUTION**
> Make sure the surfaces you lean against during your labour circuit can support your weight.

91 Supported squat against the wall

These positions help engage the muscles of the abdomen and the lower back to assist uterine contractions during labour. They also make full use of gravity to open the cervix effectively as well as to alleviate pain, particularly in the lower back. To conserve your energy, lean against the wall with your elbows resting on a windowsill, and a stool in position in case you need to sit down.

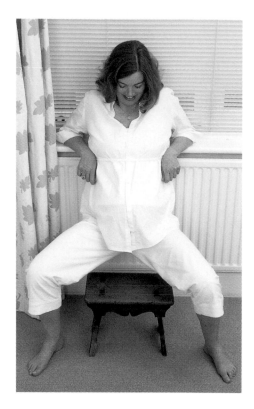

▷ **1** Stand with your legs a comfortable width apart. Now adjust your position until your back is supported by the wall as you bend your knees in a semi-squat position.

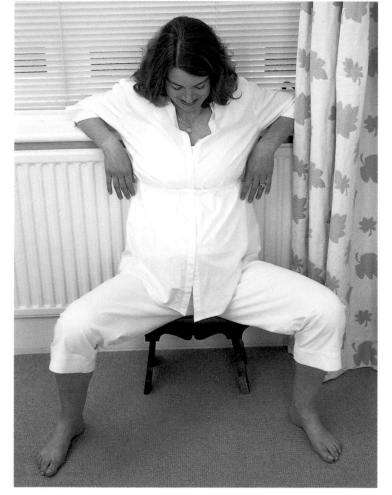

◁ **2** If this position puts too much strain on your thighs and legs, or you already need to sit down to breathe through regular contractions, lower yourself down the wall until you are sitting on the stool, still with your legs apart. Make sure that your back is upright against the wall.

92 Standing poses during labour

After squatting for a while, stand up and practise the Pink Panther Strides (79) and Hip Drops (80). When you feel a contraction starting, try these supported standing poses as they are an effective way of facilitating the descent of your baby's head. You may prefer to press down on a chest of drawers or counter with your hands rather than against the wall, but in the same standing position. Circling your hips rhythmically can feel very soothing.

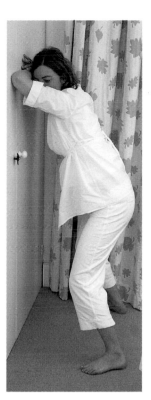

◁ **1** Face a wall and lean against it. Bend your knees and press against the wall with your forearms, resting your head on top of your joined hands.

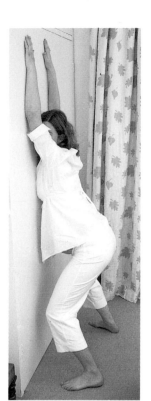

◁ **2** Then, keeping your forearms in the same place, bend your knees and let your hips drop down on an out breath. "Hang" in this position and breathe deeply, focusing on the out breaths.

93 Supported kneeling

Supported kneeling is a favourite labour position for many women and can provide you with periods of active rest during your labour. It can also be a good birthing position. It is important to adjust the position of your knees so that they are not too wide apart for comfort. Take time to install yourself in such a way that your spine is extended as much as possible while the shoulders remain relaxed. Cushions or pillows can be placed under your knees and feet for greater comfort if you need them. This position is especially soothing if you experience backache during labour, particularly if your baby is lying in a posterior position – that is, with his or her back to your back. Change position again after 15–20 minutes.

▷ **1** Use a beanbag or exercise ball to really stretch your back during labour. A ball is excellent as you can move back and forth very slightly, which is highly soothing. Hug the ball and rest your head on your arms to keep your neck comfortable.

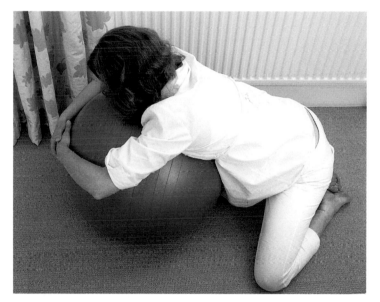

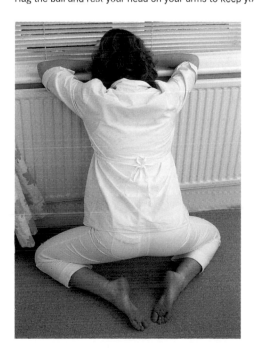

◁ **2** Use a windowsill or high bed if you prefer a more upright position. Support yourself with your forearms and make sure your neck and shoulders are relaxed.

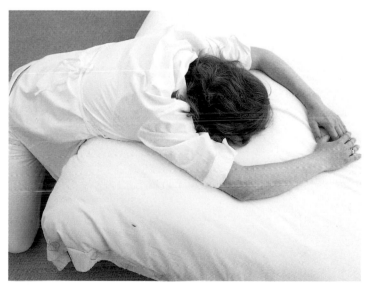

△ **3** Kneeling over a low bed with your arms above your head gives your shoulders a particularly good stretch.

Yoga breathing for labour

Many of the complications of labour arise from physical exhaustion, often made worse by lack of sleep, so you need plenty of deep rest as the birth approaches. Conserving your energy is also a priority from the moment you discover that labour is starting, and the best way to achieve this is through deep breathing that follows the rhythm of your contractions. Taking a sip of water after each contraction is helpful too. When you are fully dilated, the breath takes on another role by helping you to give birth with minimal strain.

breathe out to welcome the contractions, then let them go

In the first stage of labour, most women have contractions at intervals that gradually become shorter as the labour progresses. From the very beginning, your most important task is to relax as much as possible between the contractions and to avoid dissipating your energy, particularly by talking. Your breath out needs to be used for getting rid of tension as the contractions come and go. During each contraction, focus on breathing as deeply as you can, depending on its strength. Then start to relax again, even if only for a minute.

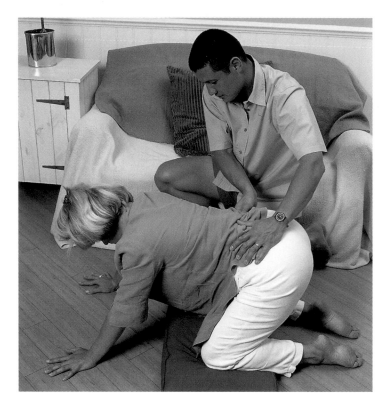

◁ Kneeling on all fours, keeping your head relaxed, can be a very effective position for grounding you and helping you to cope with backache during labour.

centring with breath during labour

Your labour circuit positions may involve your partner, who can be holding you or massaging you, or you may prefer to labour on your own, drawing deeply upon your inner resources. Whichever way is best for you, the ebb and flow of your breath can help you to remain centred through awareness of the flow of breath – both during and between your contractions. You will find that breathing is your most powerful tool for surfing the contractions rather than attempting to resist them. After any conversations or medical procedures, use your breath to re-centre yourself.

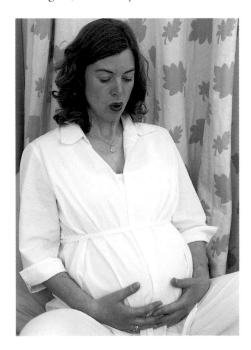

◁ Each time you feel a contraction on its way, breathe out deeply. This allows you to welcome it with relaxed muscles, and this, in turn, helps the contraction to work more effectively to open your cervix. Breathe throughout the contraction in whatever way feels best for you. When the contraction peaks, it is time to breathe out again deeply, to send it on its way and to dispel as quickly as possible the inevitable tension that results from pain.

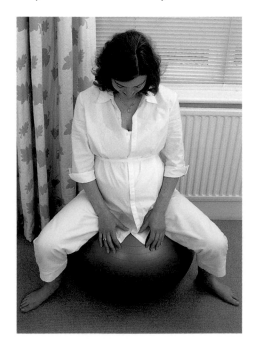

▷ Sitting astride a gym ball allows you to use gentle pelvic rocking, in time with your breath, to relax between contractions and to centre yourself once more.

breathing for birthing

The second stage of labour begins when your midwife confirms that the birth passage is fully open and ready for your baby to pass through. You may already be feeling a strong urge to push your baby out, or you may feel nothing at all. Every woman is different. The two priorities in all cases, however, are to relax as deeply as possible to make space for the baby, and to relax all the muscles of the pelvis, particularly those in the buttocks, for birthing.

When it comes to breathing, voicing your breath out, on any note that feels good to you at the time, helps the abdominal muscles to work together with the powerful bearing down contractions. The longer that you can extend the breath out, the farther your baby is able to move down the birth passage during one contraction. Engage your inner pelvic muscles on your out breath, pushing from within. Try to keep your facial muscles, and the rest of your body, as relaxed as possible as you do this, to lessen the strain.

Your midwife will guide you as to when, or if, you should breathe lightly – as if you were blowing on hot soup. This need arises if you have to hold back and wait for your perineum to stretch as the baby's head crowns. By blowing lightly, you are disengaging your abdominal muscles from your breathing and so weakening the impact of the uterine contractions.

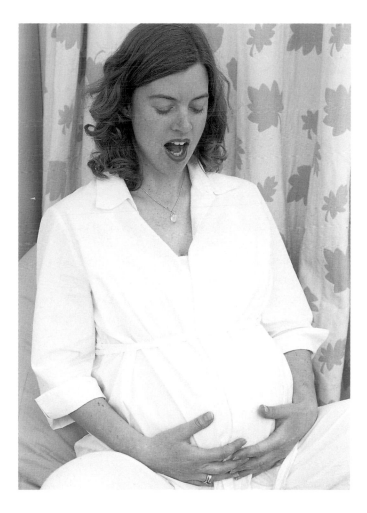

◁ Voice your breath out with a "Haaa!" sound deep into your lower abdomen. Extend it for as long as you can to increase the pressure of your contracting uterus on your baby's body as he or she moves down the birth canal.

91

31+ weeks

Gravity, centring and a voiced breath out can be combined in a powerful yet light action to push your baby out. Let awareness of your baby guide your breathing. Breathing your baby out into the world is a loving action that is open to most women and brings many possible long-term benefits to both mothers and babies. Even if medical intervention is necessary during your labour, breathing and relaxing with yoga will facilitate any birth process.

breathing to deliver the placenta

To deliver the placenta after the baby is born, use the same breathing that you employed for the birthing.

Zoë's story

Mine was a highly positive birthing experience – due to my husband's very vocal encouragement and essential breathing advice from Françoise. Having attended a yoga class throughout my pregnancy, I felt well-prepared, but when contractions suddenly started on my due date, I was taken by surprise by the strong back discomfort. I stayed at home for as long as possible with my husband and friend, timing contractions and pushing on my back to relieve the pain.

When I arrived at the hospital, my friend and husband arranged my pillows, sat me on my birthing ball and set up my specially chosen music. I started to meditate, breathing through the contractions. After a long labour, where the contractions hit me hard, and I became rather frustrated by watching the head bob back and forth for a couple of hours, I heard the word "episiotomy" from my midwife and with one contraction focused on my breathing and pushed five times to deliver my wonderful daughter, Kira.

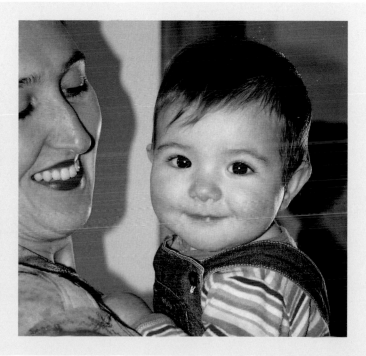

Yoga and birth positions with a partner

For many thousands of years, women in all cultures have given birth in positions that make use of gravity, although for much of the last century, Western hospitals tended to encourage women to give birth on their backs. The advantages of not lying flat on your back for giving birth have now been recognized and currently women are encouraged to sit up, or to lie on their side, for delivery on hospital beds. This is a step forward, although here we present further birthing positions that allow you to be more active still. If you have practised yoga regularly during your pregnancy, these positions should feel both familiar and comfortable. Supported standing in a semi-squat, supported squatting and variations on kneeling are all possible options that you can try out beforehand to discover which one feels best for you. Some women consistently favour a leaning-forward position while others prefer to lean back. Supported birth positions also mean that partners can be actively helpful and closely associated with the birth of their baby. In this book we refer to a male partner, but of course you can enlist the help of a female friend.

94 Birthing: supported standing positions with partner

The supporting partner must be confident that his back is strong. He leans against a wall with his feet a little away from the base of the wall and his knees slightly bent to ensure a strong bracing position. Stand as close as possible to your partner. You must feel able to let go completely, trusting that your partner's back is pressing against the wall and that he can take your weight safely during contractions. Both of you should relax between contractions.

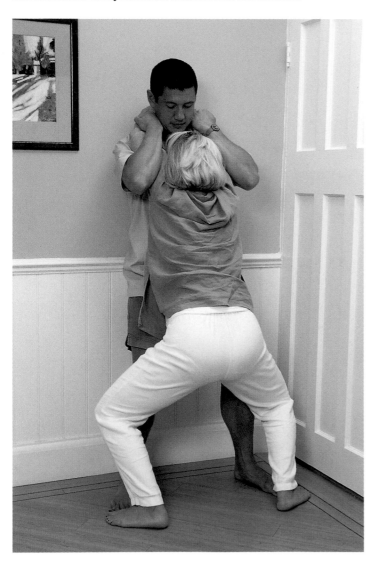

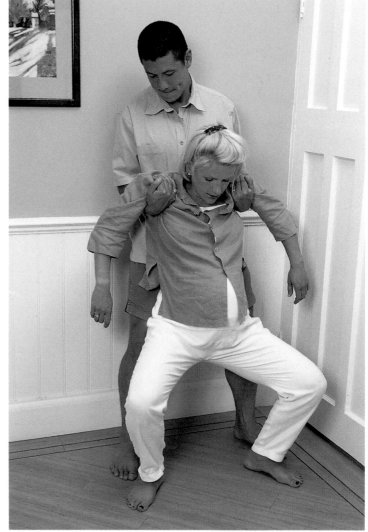

△ **First position** Face your partner and link your arms around his neck. Bend your knees and let yourself hang down.

△ **Second position** Stand with your back to your partner. Let him support you with his forearms under your arms while you bend your knees in a semi-squat.

95 Birthing: supported squatting positions with partner

Women who feel that they can create more space in their pelvis when they are leaning back can experiment with this position in one
of its variations. The first variation is an extension of the standing semi-squat, which can also be used with a birthing stool.

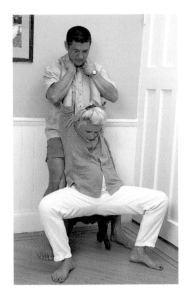 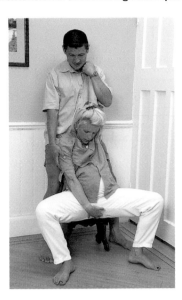 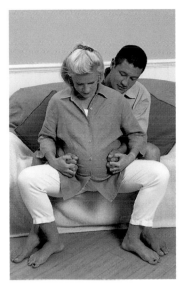 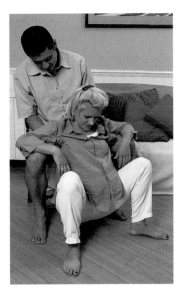

△ **First variation** 1 Use the support of a low stool so that you can squat easily while hanging from your partner's shoulders.

△ 2 During the final birthing contractions, touching your baby's crown can help you to pace and centre your breathing.

△ **Second variation** Your partner sits behind you on a sofa or wide chair while you sit on the edge, between his knees. Holding hands helps you both to centre your breathing in close harmony with each other.

△ **Third variation** Your partner sits on a chair with his legs apart and his back straight, supporting you under your arms as you drop into a wide squat. Adjust the position of your feet so you are as straight and relaxed as possible.

96 Birthing: supported kneeling positions with partner

If you choose to spend a major part of your labour on all fours, then a supported kneeling position may be the best birthing option.
There are many variations, depending on how you choose to kneel, the angle of your back and the height at which your partner sits to
support you. Be guided by your experience as you focus awareness on your pelvic floor. Put cushions under the knees for comfort.

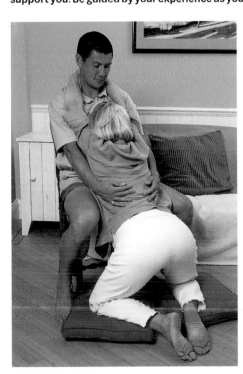 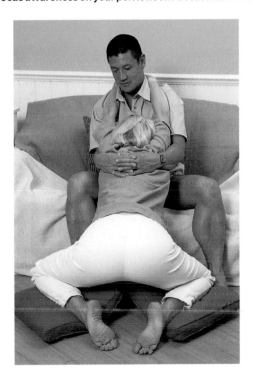 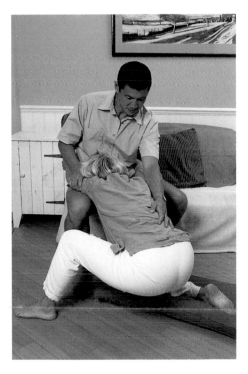

△ **1** Kneel in front of your partner, putting your arms around his neck for support. This position makes good use of gravity and relieves pain if the baby is pressing against your lower back.

△ **2** Kneel as before, but this time spread the knees wider and sit further down. The tilt of your pelvis can be modified to widen the birth passage. Let your body guide you into the best position.

△ **3** Kneel as before, but then bring one foot forward outside the knee. This position allows the widest opening in a position that may combine the advantages of both squatting and kneeling.

Medical intervention: questions and answers

• How will yoga affect whether or not I have medical intervention?
Practising yoga while pregnant gives you the best possible chance of a happy, intervention-free outcome, although complications can occur. Hope for the best possible scenario and then calmly revise your expectations should difficulties arise. If they do, yoga will still help: deep breathing and relaxation reduce stress; body-awareness helps you adjust your position effectively even when movement is restricted; and yoga helps you remain connected with your baby throughout any interventions, and in harmony with your care team.

• Do yogic techniques work when attached to a monitor?
You can adopt several active birth positions when attached to a monitor. Adjust the bed head to the most comfortable sitting position, usually around a 25° angle. When you are comfortable, bend your legs alternately for about 10 minutes, placing the sole of the foot of the bent leg against the inner thigh of the straight leg. Breathe calmly for as long as possible through contractions. Alternatively, kneel on the bed and lean against the bed head (still at a 25° angle), using pillows for support. Lastly, try resting on your side in the relaxation position, with one bent leg above the other and a pillow between your knees. Alternate between these positions every half hour or so. This creates a sense of rhythm that may provide relief from contraction pain.

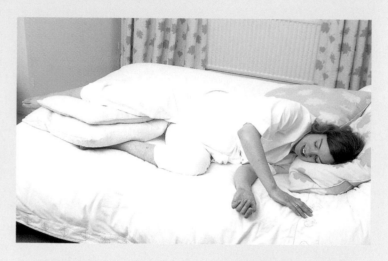

△ **Try to remember this position just in case you are attached to a monitor at some point during the birthing. It is also recommended if you have had epidural analgesia.**

• How would I cope with instrumental delivery?
Ventouse or forceps deliveries can be stressful for you and your baby. Try to relax as deeply as possible to eliminate all resistance. Even if you have an epidural analgesic, mental surrender can make a big difference and facilitate delivery. Try to remain connected to your baby during this procedure and take extra time for bonding as soon as your baby is born.

• Can yoga help in the case of an emergency section?
During this operation, you will be anaesthetized but remain conscious. Remember that your baby will be with you very soon. Use deep breathing, focusing on the breath out, to centre yourself and to minimize the overall impact of this operation on your nervous system. Relax with each breath out and surrender yourself to the process. Visualize yourself holding your baby's hand from inside as you are prepared for theatre. The deeper that you are able to relax, the less morphine you may need after the operation, and therefore, the more alert you will be to welcome your new baby into the world.

• What happens if the placenta's delivery is delayed?
You can help to trigger the uterine contractions needed for the expulsion of the placenta, so resume your labour circuit. The yoga exercises will help here, as they did for the birth.

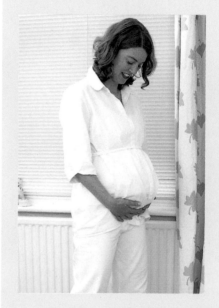

◁ **Good breathing practices help greatly throughout pregnancy and labour. Deep down-breaths can also be used to encourage the contractions needed to deliver the placenta.**

A sample practice for late pregnancy

1 ▽ Centring into the earth (70)

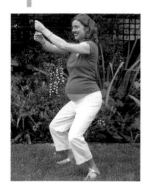

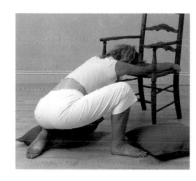

2 △ Perineal stretch with chair (77)

3 ▽ Supported kneeling (93)

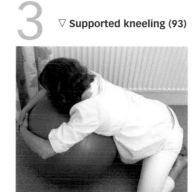

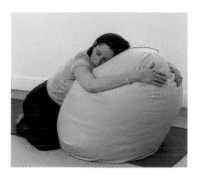

4 △ Hugging rest (72)

Useful addresses and thanks

GETTING IN TOUCH

Yoga classes and training courses for conception, pregnancy, birth and beyond:
Birthlight
P.O.Box 148, Cambridge CB4 2GB, UK
Tel 01223 362288
www.birthlight.com
Email: enquiries@birthlight.com
Birthlight has a national and international network of specially trained pre- and postnatal yoga teachers.

General yoga classes, with fully trained teachers:
The British Wheel of Yoga
25 Jermyn Street, Sleaford, Lincolnshire
NG34 7RU, UK
Tel 01529 306 851
www.bwy.org.uk
Email: office@bwy.org.uk

General health advice for prospective parents:
Foresight
Association for the Promotion of Pre-conceptual Care
28 The Paddock, Godalming, Surrey
GU7 1XD, UK
Tel 01483 427839/419468
www.foresight-preconception.org.uk

Information and referral to support groups:
National Childbirth Trust (NCT)
Alexandra House, Oldham Terrace, Acton, London W3 6NH, UK
Tel 0870 7703236
www.nctpregnancyandbabycare.com

Information and advice on prenatal matters:
Organization for Prenatal Education
Tel 01892 784381
Email: contact@ope.org.uk

AUSTRALIA: *Umbrella organization for information and classes:*
Childbirth Education Association of Australia
P.O.Box 413, Hurstville BC, NSW, 1481
Australia
Tel (02) 9580 0399
www.cea-nsw.com.au
Email: info@cea-nsw.com.au

USA: *Contact network for childbirth information (including International Alliance of Midwives):*
Midwifery Today, Inc.
P.O.Box 2672-350, Eugene OR 97402, USA
Tel (USA) 541 344 7438
www.midwiferytoday.com
Email: inquiries@midwiferytoday.com

AUTHORS' ACKNOWLEDGEMENTS:

Doriel Hall: I would like to thank everyone involved, especially my colleague Françoise, and Bel Gibbs for the use of her lovely home and for all the help from her friends.
Françoise Freedman: My thanks go first of all to many yoga teachers and to all the Birthlight mothers who have helped me develop and refine the approach presented in this book over half a lifetime. Among them is Sally Lomas, radiant in this book with her fourth baby Fyn, who has become a leading Birthlight tutor and friend. Thanks to very dear Doriel Hall, with whom friendship has deepened through our collaboration as co-authors. Thanks also to Debra Mayhew for her painstaking editing, done in a skilful, sensitive and relaxed style that left all involved happy with their jobs, and to Ann Kay for her diligent completion of the book. Thanks to all those people who have supported me in making this yoga more accessible to mothers-to-be, particularly Rhea Quien, Margaret Adey, Elizabeth de Michelis and the Trustees of Birthlight. Thanks to Robin Monro for giving Perinatal Yoga importance and recognition at the Yoga Biomedical Trust long before it became common practice. Thanks to Andrea Wilson and Uma Dinsmore, among many special co-teachers, for their unfailing dedication to yoga for mothers. My warmest thanks are to my whole family for their love and inspiration. Thanks also to the Amazonian women who showed me the midwifery and mothering of their world. It is my wish that the yoga in this book may be a bridge between them and the magical work of midwives and Doulas in the West in order to empower women in pregnancy and birth.

Thank you to the models
The publishers would like to thank all the models, who are such good ambassadors for the positive benefits of yoga. The incredible energy and vitality shown by even the most heavily pregnant models was an inspiration. Our models: Margaret Bishop, Moira Bogue, Simon Bower, Karen Brown, Anna Cuirleo, Laura Dymock, Bel Gibbs, Sally Lomas with mother Diana Lomas and son Aron (5), Antony Malvasi, Zoë Moghadas, Rachel Moore, Angela Nutt and daughter Alabama (19 months), Celine Smith, Annie and Bob Taylor, Jane Tudman, Lucie Witney. Also MOT Models agency and their models Liza Licence and Elizabeth Tarrant.

Thanks also to Elizabeth Wright for her photograph of Zoë and daughter Kira for "Zoë's Story", and to Pat Coward for the index.

Index

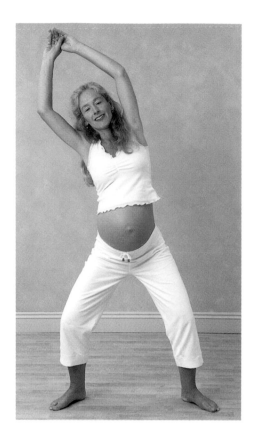

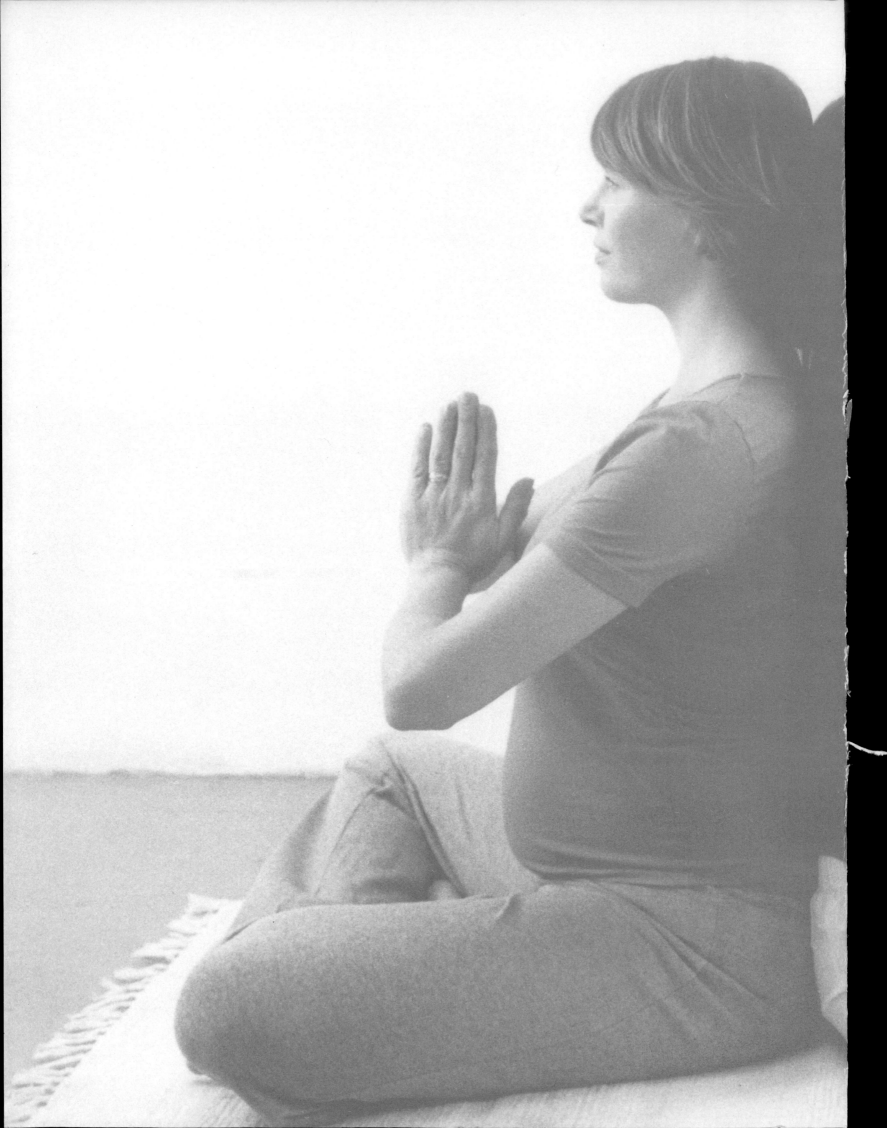